D1562838

The Biology of Homosexuality

Oxford Series in Behavioral Neuroendocrinology

Editors
Gregory F. Ball, Johns Hopkins University
Jacques Balthazart, University of Liège
Randy J. Nelson, Ohio State University

Luis Miguel Garcia-Segura, *Hormones and Brain Plasticity*
Jacques Balthazart, *The Biology of Homosexuality*

The Biology of Homosexuality

JACQUES BALTHAZART, PhD

GIGA Neurosciences
University of Liège, Belgium

OXFORD
UNIVERSITY PRESS

OXFORD
UNIVERSITY PRESS

Published in the United States of America by Oxford University Press, Inc.,
198 Madison Avenue, New York, NY, 10016
United States of America

Oxford University Press, Inc. publishes works that further Oxford University's objective
of excellence in research, scholarship, and education

Oxford is a registered trade mark of Oxford University Press in the UK and in certain other countries

Library of Congress Cataloging-in-Publication Data

Balthazart, J. (Jacques), 1949-
  The biology of homosexuality / Jacques Balthazart.
    p. cm.
  Includes bibliographical references and index.
  ISBN 978-0-19-983882-0 (hardback)
  1. Homosexuality. 2. Sexual orientation. I. Title.
  HQ76.25.B35 2011
  306.76'6—dc23   2011036460

1 3 5 7 9 10 8 6 4 2

Typeset in Minion Pro
Printed on acid-free paper
Printed in the United States of America

ACKNOWLEDGMENTS

I would like to thank my wife, Claire, and my daughter-in-law, Nathalie, not only for their constant support but also for the constructive criticism that they provided at multiple stages during the writing of this book. This book would not have been written without their help.

At Oxford University Press, Catharine Carlin initiated this project and Joan Bossert brought it to completion. They both played a key role in publication. Steve Holtje greatly improved my original translation of the text from French to English, and I would like to thank him for his essential contribution.

Finally several members in my laboratory, in particular, Dr. Charlotte A. Cornil, provided useful critiques and suggestions at various stages of writing. Thank you very much.

CONTENTS

INTRODUCTION: WHY THIS BOOK?

The attitude of Western societies toward homosexuals has changed considerably over the centuries. The very tolerant attitude that prevailed for much of Greco-Roman antiquity and the Middle Ages was followed by a time of greater intolerance largely inspired by changes in Judeo-Christian thinking. Homosexuality was then seen as a stigma or a perversion that should be fought and treated like a disease. Later, various schools of thought inspired by Freudian or post-Freudian theories attributed a critical role in the development of homosexuality to the attitude of parents toward their young children.

Based on scientific results accumulated over the past few decades, I believe, in contrast, that the origin of homosexuality must be sought in the biology of individuals who express this particular sexual orientation rather than in the behavior of their parents or in the life choices made by individuals during their development. It is the purpose of this book to summarize the arguments that support this conclusion. Neither the education that parents provided nor their own behavior (e.g., absent father or dominant mother) induced the homosexuality of their child. In this conceptual framework, to blame parents is irrelevant. (Please understand that the use of the word "blame" here and elsewhere in the book is not a statement that homosexuality is blameworthy, but an observation and comment on behavior in societies where stigma is attached to homosexuality.)

It is crucial to understand that for the vast majority of subjects, homosexual behavior develops independently of any kind of choice. It is even frequently in conflict with the choices that are consciously made by the individual. The discovery of their homosexual orientation is, for many adolescents, painful and only accepted gradually in their life, if ever. This undoubtedly helps to explain the so-called cases of change in sexual orientation–homosexuals who contracted a heterosexual marriage and then apparently changed their orientation. The first orientation was often the result of social pressures that the individual took decades to overcome before accepting his or her true nature. This difficulty in accepting an unexpected sexual orientation is also at the root of the increased suicide rate in the homosexual population as compared with matched heterosexual populations (Kourany, 1987; Lebson, 2002).

This reflection on the social consequences of one or the other interpretation of homosexuality does not affect our analysis of its causes. The conclusions based on evidence must of course take precedence. That said, in light of this evidence, I hope this book will help make society aware that sexual orientation is probably under the control of embryonic endocrine/genetic phenomena in which there is little room for individual choice. Therefore society needs to rethink its attitudes toward homosexuals and their parents.

Animal studies are of great support in understanding the controlling forces of sexuality. These studies demonstrate the existence in animals of neurobiological mechanisms determining the behavior and sexual orientation that seem also to be present, *mutatis mutandis*, in human studies. This experimental work, carried out in strictly controlled conditions, provides a strong support to interpret correlative studies conducted in humans, even if the details of the mechanisms involved are currently not fully understood. They probably never can be, given that it is impossible to perform most types of experiments in humans (for obvious ethical reasons) and that there is a very long latency (greater than 20 years) between the events that probably induce homo- or heterosexuality (endocrine environment of the embryo and its genetic heritage) and the identification of their effects (sexual orientation of the adult). Prospective studies are thus extremely difficult and expensive if you consider, in addition, the limited number of homosexuals who appear in the population studied. Retrospective studies are possible, but less convincing because the selection of subjects and their controls, even if they are well matched, can be skewed by unidentified factors.

For more than 35 years, I have been studying the hormonal and neural mechanisms that control the so-called instinctive behaviors (spontaneously expressed and species-specific) in animals. Much of this work has been devoted to the study of male sexual behavior, and led me to turn my attention to sex differences that are associated with this behavior. In most species, males and females indeed show different behaviors, and furthermore they mostly direct these behaviors toward the opposite sex (i.e., they show a marked sex difference in sexual orientation). These differences in behavior and its orientation are clearly controlled in animals by steroid hormones produced by the gonads.

The action of these steroids on behavior takes place mostly in the brain, particularly in some of its oldest parts from an evolutionary point of view, the hypothalamus and preoptic area. The primary goal of research in neuroendocrinology is to advance, at the basic level, our knowledge of how the brain functions. Clearly, however, the potential application of this knowledge to the human species is an issue that cannot be escaped. Is human sexual behavior under the control of testicular and ovarian hormones? And do these hormones affect the orientation of this behavior?

It is interesting that research on the neuroendocrine basis of sexual behavior in animals and humans is a discipline that has developed more in the Anglo-Saxon countries, mainly the United States and to a lesser extent Great Britain.

The bulk of the scientific literature in this area is therefore published in English. For the same reason, there are also a few English-language books devoted to the biological mechanisms that control animal or human sexuality in general, including sometimes a discussion of sexual orientation (LeVay, 1993; 1996; Strong & DeVault, 1997; Rosenzweig et al., 2004; LeVay & Valente, 2006; Agmo, 2007).

However, there is not, to my knowledge, a simple description of the biological mechanisms that are involved in the determination of sexual orientation in animals and also presumably in humans. By showing herein that the sexual orientation of a subject is controlled by a set of biological and environmental factors, I hope to provide that book. This text was originally written and published in French in early February 2010. While its English version was being prepared, another book written by Simon LeVay was published that also focuses on the biological bases of human homosexuality (*Gay, Straight, and the Reason Why*, Oxford University Press, 2010). Although much of the experimental evidence presented in LeVay's book is also discussed here, these two books differ in their overall approach. LeVay starts from the notion of sexual orientation in humans and discusses this orientation based on human studies largely, using animal studies mainly to support conclusions derived from observations in humans. In contrast, the present text starts from the animal work that is the focus of my scientific research and in a second step analyzes how this animal work potentially applies to humans. It's quite interesting that while these two books start from different premises, they reach the exact same conclusion, that is, that homosexuality in humans is to a very large extent, if not exclusively, determined by biological factors acting prenatally or soon after birth and that the social or educational environment plays at best a subsidiary role in this determinism. The conjunction of these two books thus strongly reinforces the general conclusion presented in the following pages.

It must also be noted that while describing the experimental support of this thesis, the book will focus on more than just homosexuality, as the context in which biological factors act produces multiple results. Ignoring the nonhomosexual results of the process would present an incomplete, context-free picture of the factors at work. Thus, even readers not particularly interested in homosexuality will find this book a useful guide to the biological bases of sexual orientation. Understanding the roots of homosexuality requires also investigating the bases of heterosexuality, since both forms of sexual orientation only represent the two extremes of a continuum called sexual orientation. This question is then of interest to everyone. I will also note in advance that because male homosexuality is more clear-cut than female homosexuality and its biological origins are better documented, at times it will dominate the discussion. This is merely an unfortunate result of where our current scientific understanding lies and nothing more. This book presents as balanced a portrait as possible, and no slight or judgment is intended.

Scientists reading this book will think, "We have heard all this before." Certainly the content of this book is not scientifically revolutionary; it has been known for at least a decade, though over that time more evidence has continued to pile up. But somehow that information has either not made its way into the world outside the laboratory or has not been presented in a sufficiently definitive manner to affect the general population's views on the matter (with the exception of the book of Simon LeVay mentioned in the preceding paragraph [LeVay, 2010]). Scientists are thus not the only audience for which this book is intended. This is a book also for laymen, but it contains enough science that rather than just being told "X is true," they are shown why it's true in a way that I hope will give them a genuine understanding of the subject, not just an opinion. In this respect, this book can thus also be used by scientists and teachers for their seminars or advanced courses on sexuality. However, if they wish, readers can skip over the more hardcore science in Chapters 3–4 and still emerge with plenty of useful knowledge. There's a glossary at the end that will help those readers navigate the later chapters.

Of course, presenting a mass of facts without a guiding organization would result in a mere collection of lab reports, not a book. Some will say this book advocates a specific position rather than letting readers draw their own conclusions. I arrived at this position because the scientific facts led there. They also led Simon LeVay to this same conclusion, and that's why this book leads readers to the same place.

The Biology of Homosexuality

1

Sexuality 101

The Basics

THE FOUR DIMENSIONS OF HUMAN SEXUALITY

Human sexuality is a complex and multidimensional phenomenon that covers various aspects of behavior and personality. Four dimensions that are partly but not completely independent can be distinguished: (1) the type of specific action patterns that are produced by the individual (performance) and the motivation underlying the expression of these behaviors; (2) the orientation of the behavior and of sexual fantasies associated with it (sexual orientation); (3) the sexual identity that the individual believes he or she has; and (4) the sexual role that the individual plays in the society. These four dimensions are often correlated within an individual and linked to his or her physical and genetic sex, but major discrepancies may occur. In order to clarify important points of terminology, sexologists speak of **homosexuality** when the sexual orientation of an individual does not correspond to his or her physical sex (the form of his or her genitals), of **transsexuality** when the sexual identity is at odds with the physical sex, and of **transvestism** when the gender role played by an individual does not correspond to his or her physical sex. Generally speaking, the action of sex steroids and biological variables on these various components of sexuality is extremely variable.

The first aspect of human sexuality is linked to the performance of sexual acts and the motivation behind them. It has been shown in animals that this feature is sexually differentiated and controlled by steroid hormones during both development (organization) and adulthood (activation) (Chapter 3). Human *sexual behavior* is not limited to sexually differentiated motor actions. Instead of having a stereotyped mating, as is the case in rats (mounting and penetrating by the male, lordosis posture [downward arching of the spine and raising of the hips] in the female), the human species mates in a variety of positions. A position is often preferred in a given culture (the woman lying on her back, face to face with the man—the so-called "missionary position"— in Western civilization), but other positions are commonly used, and favorite positions vary from one culture to another (Nelson, 2005). Men and women do not play stereotypical roles in the sexual act, nor is there a major differ- ence between the motor acts performed by both sexes, and consequently, the animal literature on mechanisms that control dimorphism affecting this aspect of behavior has little contribution toward understanding the human species. Furthermore, there is little difference between men and women in intensity of sexual motivation. Differences in modality have been reported, but they are minor and often related to culture. This motivation, even if it is not very sexually differentiated, remains partly under the control of sex steroids in humans and animals, and I shall review the arguments that support this thesis (Chapter 7).

If the motor aspects of sexual behavior are quite similar among men and women, the three other dimensions of sexuality are highly differentiated.

Sexual orientation, a term that I prefer to sexual preference because of its neutrality in relation to the will of the individual, identifies the sex of persons to which an individual directs not only his or her behavior but also sexual fanta- sies. Most men and women are sexually attracted and excited by individuals of the opposite sex. They are heterosexual. However, there are individuals— occurring at quite a regular percentage—attracted to persons of their own sex; they are homosexual. This distinction is not absolute; following qualitative studies from Kinsey and colleagues in the late 1940s, it was recognized that all intermediaries could exist. It is considered that 3 to 10% of men are homosexu- als in all cultures irrespective of their culture's attitude vis-à-vis homosexuality. These numbers vary slightly depending on the study methods (see Chapter 2). The figures for women are less accurate, but should be of the same order of magnitude with the addition of a significant population of individuals regard- ing themselves as bisexual (attraction to women as well as men). There thus exists in all human populations a significant proportion of gays and lesbians. Although very significant, this ratio never exceeds 10%, which means that the vast majority of the general population is heterosexual. Sexual orientation is one of the behavioral traits most differentiated between men and women that has been identified.

Regardless of which sex is found interesting or exciting, each human being is also confident of belonging to one sex, male or female. This conviction is unchangeable, and it often seems to develop during early childhood. Most people have a **sexual identity** that matches their genitalia, although a small number of people are convinced to the contrary and believe themselves "to be born in a body that does not correspond to their gender." They are called transsexuals by sexologists. This gender identity is already apparent in early childhood and, contrary to what was thought until recently, it is usually difficult or impossible to change it later (see the story of John/Joan, Chapter 2). Clinical data suggest that the organization of sexual identity could be controlled by prenatal sex steroids. This idea is difficult to assess, in part because there is no animal model for studying sexual identity. It is impossible to ask an animal, whatever its species, to what sex it belongs. In addition to communication difficulties associated with such an undertaking, this would imply that the animal is aware of its own body and sex, which is far from proved even though recent research daily shows new sophisticated cognitive skills not only among primates but also in species more distant from humans, such as dolphins and even birds such as parrots and corvids (a family including crows and jays).

The fourth and last dimension of human sexuality concerns the role played by an individual in society. This **gender role** is deeply influenced by the structure of the society in which the individual lives, even if prenatal hormonal influences also seem to play a role (see Chapter 2). Thus, housework tasks were typically performed by women in Western Europe until the First World War, but are now widely shared by men and women. Farm work tasks also are typically male or female depending on the human group. It would probably be futile to search for biological bases for this type of sexual difference, even if sociobiology suggests that selective pressures acting on our ancestors may have selectively adjusted men and women for various jobs (this idea is broadly contested). Other aspects of the gender role (play behavior during childhood, hobbies, etc.), however, may be influenced by prenatal factors.

The four dimensions of human sexuality that I have distinguished are correlated and in agreement with each other in the majority of individuals. This correlation can be expected both on the basis of coordinated learning that affects these different features and on the basis of a prenatal hormonal environment that plays a role in their organization. However, it is important to distinguish them clearly, because these dimensions may be exceptionally discordant. In particular, it is critical to distinguish between orientation and gender identity. A transsexual man who thinks he in fact is a woman may be sexually attracted by men or by women; sexual identity does not determine sexual attraction, or vice versa. This orientation becomes difficult to classify because it will depend on the sex of reference considered (physical/genetic and genital sex, or sex corresponding to sexual identity). For example, a transsexual man-to-woman attracted to men is gay if one refers to his physical sex but hetero-sexual if we consider his sexual identity.

For various technical and ethical reasons, the experimental analysis of the neurobiological bases of sexuality is difficult for humans, and it must often be limited to the study of clinical cases. The interpretation of these data usually remains problematic because they are essentially correlative (existence of a rela-tionship between a behavioral character and hormonal changes, for example). It is impossible to be certain that the observed correlations are due to the effects of one variable or the other. The confirmation of these interpretations can therefore only come indirectly from comparison with true causal studies per-formed on animals.

Most animal studies devoted to sex differences affecting sexual behavior have unfortunately focused on the differences in the type of behavior patterns that are expressed by the two sexes. These studies are therefore of little interest for the understanding of human behavior, in which patterns of behavior expressed by men and women during sexual interactions show little or no dif-ference. More recently, studies of sexual orientation were also started in ani-mals, and we will see that these studies provide important insights into the origins of human homo- or heterosexuality. The other two dimensions of sexu-ality, sexual identity and role, are specific to humans and cannot be studied in animal models.

It is important to distinguish three aspects of homosexuality, namely the expression of homosexual behavior(s), the homosexual attraction, and finally the recognition/acceptance of this attraction vis-à-vis society. Expressing occa-sional or even regular sexual behavior directed toward an individual of the same sex is found frequently in various animal species (Bagemihl, 1999; Sommer & Vasey, 2006; Poianni, 2010). This is generally associated with conditions under which partners of the opposite sex are not (easily) available. One can point to captive animals (zoo, farm), to animal societies where a few dominant males monopolize all females and dominated males are prevented from mating with them, or to groups of animals where the sex ratio (relative number of males and females) is highly skewed so that many individuals cannot find a partner of the opposite sex. In all these cases, homosexual behavior will often disappear quickly when partners of the opposite sex become available (Sommer & Vasey, 2006; Poianni, 2010).

The same is true in humans: there is a fairly regular basis of homosexual behavior in circumstances where partners of the opposite sex are not available, such as in prisons or single-sex institutions of learning. I also discuss in this book so-called primitive societies where homosexual relations are the norm among teenagers, even encouraged, because access to girls is forbidden before marriage (Chapter 2). In all these circumstances, it was observed that homosexual behaviors regress or disappear when opposite-sex partners become available, so there is not preferential homosexual attraction in these cases. The homosexual activity is simply an outlet for sexual motivation without necessarily being preferred to heterosexual activity.

The preferential or exclusive attraction to partners of the same sex is in contrast a largely human characteristic that does not occur frequently in animals but can be induced by changes in the embryonic hormonal environment or by injury to a specific area of the brain. Such spontaneous exclusive homosexual attraction has been identified in certain populations of sheep (Chapter 4). This is the preferential or exclusive attraction to individuals of the same sex that I am talking about mainly in this book. I will show that this attraction is dependent, at least in part, on prenatal biological phenomena that are largely beyond the will of the concerned individual.

The open display in society of this homosexual attraction is the third and last aspect to be considered independently. It is clear that this public revelation can only follow prior personal acceptance of homosexual orientation. Its public disclosure ("coming out") is, however, a conscious act that largely depends on the willingness of the person. This willingness interacts with the greater or lesser tolerance of those around him or her, which will facilitate or complicate the process. Many homosexuals, including some very famous ones (to name a few, writer Gertrude Stein, blues singer Alberta Hunter, and tennis player Billie Jean King among women; writer Marcel Proust, composer Peter Ilyich Tchaikovsky, and actor Rock Hudson among men), have historically lived with their sexual orientation in a more or less hidden condition.

The public disclosure and recognition of homosexuality are largely influenced by social context and the willingness of the individual. However, homosexual orientation develops in a distinctively independent manner from the will of the individual, under the influence of biological factors that act mostly during embryonic life. That is the point of this book.

Note, though, that I am well aware that homosexuality (and sexual orientation in general) is a complex phenomenon that is probably not the result of a single cause. In addition, male and female homosexuality may have different explanations, at least in part. Finally, within the same sex, it is likely that different reasons or causes, or a combination thereof, can induce and thus explain the homosexual orientation. I put forward in this book all the work showing that at least a part of male and female homosexuality has a biological origin related to endocrine or genetic factors. This does not preclude a potential contribution of social influences and education, or conscious choices made in adulthood. But though many popular books claim to explain homosexuality on the basis of educational or social factors, the currently available scientific studies show little or no influence of education on the development of sexual orientation.

I shall adopt in this book a fully deterministic attitude, assuming that a same cause always produces the same effects. However, in biology and even in psychology, causes are often multiple and frequently combined to create an effect. It is therefore, in some cases, difficult or sometimes impossible to formally identify the underlying causes of a given phenomenon. This does not, however, bring into question the deterministic principle. Accepting that events or behaviors are not determined would lead a scientist to admit that the causal study of behavior is impossible. This can be justified in some areas of mental activity, such as religious belief, but not in science. This being said, religion and science are not contradictory; they simply represent different approaches to reality that are not comparable and cannot be reduced to one another. I believe that animal and human behavior can in most of its aspects be analyzed by the objective methods of Cartesian deductive logic.

Multiple genetic, hormonal and environmental factors interact to modulate and control individual human behavior. They include the structure of the genome and its individual variations; and the social, hormonal, and environmental stimuli to which the individual is exposed throughout his or her lifetime. In most cases it is thus impossible to attribute a behavior to a single specific cause. A given cause only contributes to the explanation of a behavior for a certain percentage of the observed variance. We must use statistics and probabilities to draw firm conclusions. This does not, however, contradict the concept of determinism.

MALE AND FEMALE HOMOSEXUALITY: HOMOSEXUALITY AND BISEXUALITY

Because more or less negative or even hostile reactions to homosexuality and bisexuality are present in most societies, the incidence of homosexuality and bisexuality has always been difficult to assess. The first published attempt at objective quantification was that of sexologist Alfred Kinsey and his collaborators in the mid-twentieth century (Kinsey et al., 1948). Kinsey concluded that about 10% of men are exclusively or nearly exclusively homosexual, while the corresponding proportion was about 1.5% among women (Kinsey et al., 1953).

Studies based on approaches ensuring absolute anonymity of respondents have led to slightly different estimates. For example, in 2005, the National Health Statistics Center of the Centers for Disease Control and Prevention

(NHSC) used a self-administered survey and reported that 7.1% of men and 13.6% of women feel sexual attraction for people of their own sex (Mosher et al., 2005). But only 1.5% of men and 0.7% of women reported exclusively homosexual attraction (see Figure 1.1). These data could be an underestimate, but it is likely that they are closer to reality than the estimates of Kinsey and colleagues, given the greater precautions taken to ensure the objectivity of the responses of subjects and the representativeness of the analyzed samples. Despite the biases that are potentially present in all such studies, reported percentages of homosexuality in all societies studied mostly vary between 2 and 10% (Chapter 2). While slight variations are observed, these percentages are relatively similar in two studies conducted more than 50 years apart. The attitude of society toward homosexuals has changed profoundly in this period; based on that, we would expect an increase in their relative numbers, but the opposite is observed in all cases for men. This stability obviously suggests questions about the mechanisms that lead to such a consistency.

The work of Kinsey and colleagues used a seven-point scale to characterize the sexual orientation of individuals ranging from zero (totally heterosexual) to six (exclusively homosexual). The latest NHSC research is based on a five-point scale that seems to provide more reproducible results. As shown in Figure 1.1,

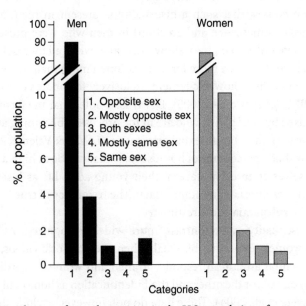

Figure 1.1 Distribution of sexual attraction in the U.S. population of men and women aged 18 to 44 years (according to data in Mosher et al., 2005). Note that the vertical axis is interrupted between 10 and 80% (angled lines) in order to permit visualization of detail in the low range of this axis.

the vast majority of individuals, for both sexes, has a preferential or exclusive attraction to individuals of the opposite sex.

It is interesting that the curve describing the distribution of sexual orientations is different for men and women. For men, there is clearly a bimodal distribution that has two peaks at the extremes (strictly heterosexual and strictly homosexual), while among women there is instead a gradual decrease of percentages when moving from an exclusively heterosexual to exclusively homosexual orientation. Thus, the categories homosexual and heterosexual describe relatively separated populations in men, while this distinction is more subtle in women.

Correspondingly, the stability of sexual orientation would be greater in men than in women. Longitudinal studies show that bisexual women or women with a nonexclusive preference for one sex more frequently change their sexual orientation than men. Sexual orientation is, however, generally stable over time. Only a small percentage of subjects change during their lifetime.

Finally, bisexuality, defined as the existence of any degree of attraction for both sexes, seems to be more common than strict homosexuality. This broad definition of bisexuality, however, includes a large number of individuals who are attracted much more to one sex than the other. If we define a more restrictive bisexuality as an attraction more or less equal to subjects of both sexes, it is then observed much more rarely in men than in women. Some sexologists even contest that such a bisexuality is present in men. Measures of genital arousal (tumescence and erection) in men who were presented erotic pictures of men and women have shown that men who call themselves bisexual show genital arousal much more for one sex (often men) than the other (Rieger et al., 2005) and often show excitement exclusively for photos of male subjects (Freund, 1974) (Rieger et al., 2005). LeVay also notes that the term *bisexual* is frequently used by young men who are in the process of becoming aware of and publicly revealing their homosexual orientation (LeVay & Valente, 2006). Some studies show that a percentage of homosexuals that can be as high as 40% identified themselves at an early stage of their young adult life as bisexual before describing themselves later as homosexual. The frequency of true bisexuality in men could be substantially overestimated.

Female bisexuality is, in contrast, more widely recognized. At the genital level, most women are in fact bisexual; when shown erotic videos, their reactions show genital arousal in response to men and women regardless of their attraction to one sex or the other and their identification as homo-, bi-, or heterosexual (Chivers et al., 2004). These data do not, however, exclude the existence of exclusive homo- or heterosexuality among women. They only show that the physiological genital arousal can be (partly) independent of verbal statements of sexual attraction.

Finally, one must clearly distinguish between sexual physical attraction and the desire for emotional intimacy. These two aspects of the human personality are not always correlated, and persons (usually women) physically attracted by one sex may fall in love with people of the opposite sex or of both sexes. This dichotomy obviously complicates the definition of bisexuality. It particularly affects women in Western cultures, but in other cultures there are also passionate friendships between heterosexual men that do not include any physical sexual element (Nardi, 1992, in LeVay & Valente, 2006, p. 228).

2

Sexuality and Sexual Orientation

Learning or Biology?

EDUCATION AND ENVIRONMENT CANNOT SUFFICE TO EXPLAIN HOMOSEXUALITY

In this chapter I briefly review the various theories that have been advanced to explain homosexuality from an environmental perspective and show why these theories, although they are still widespread, are not satisfactory and are not supported by experimental evidence. [Interested readers may usefully refer to more comprehensive books on the subject (e.g., LeVay, 1996).] Remember that the arguments presented here concern exclusively homosexual orientation as defined in Chapter 1: exclusive or preferential sexual attraction for persons of the same sex. The expression of homosexual behavior when heterosexual partners are not available and public disclosure of homosexual orientation (coming out) are, in contrast, deeply influenced by an individual's environment, previous history, learning, and education.

EFFECT OF EARLY SEXUAL EXPERIENCES

Some have argued that sexual orientation is largely determined by early life experiences. This early experience could be traumatic and aversive (e.g., rape of a girl by a man) and induce a repulsion for members of the same sex as the perpetrator of the assault: the girl would become disgusted with men and sexually attracted by women, therefore being a lesbian. Alternatively, the early experience could be attractive and, in this case, lead to a sexual orientation toward members of the sex having played an active role in this experiment. One could imagine a young boy, involved in a pedophile relationship with an adult male, experiencing pleasure and consequently developing as homosexual and finding sexual pleasure in the company of men (Churchill, 1967; Cameron & Cameron, 1995). This theory is similar to the concept of impregnation ("imprinting") developed by ethologists, which proposes that the first experiences of a young animal induce lifelong preferences (Lorenz, 1937; Lorenz, 1950).

This interpretation does not, however, take into account a number of observations. There are many societies where homosexual relations are the rule among adolescent boys [e.g., some cultures in New Guinea, see (Diamond, 1993)]. This social structure favoring homosexuality in adolescents is implemented in a more or less organized way in order to preserve the virginity of girls before marriage. The homosexual relationship of young boys with an adult male would also play an initiatory role. Various anthropological studies have clearly established that in adulthood, the percentage of men in these societies who persist in a homosexual orientation is not above the average found in other societies that forbid juvenile homosexuality. The first sexual experiences of these young boys do not seem to significantly affect their future sexual orientation (see Table 2.1) (Diamond, 1993).

Table 2-1. PERCENTAGES OF HOMOSEXUAL MEN
IN DIFFERENT SOCIETIES

Great Britain	5.0–9.0
Japan	5.8
The Netherlands	7.8
USA	4.8
Phillipines*	2.0
Pilau (Malaysia)*	4.7
Thailand*	3.6
Mean	**4.8–5.4**

Table 2.1: The table lists average percentage of male homosexuality in several European, North American and Asian countries that differ widely in their attitude toward homosexual orientation. The 3 countries whose name is followed by an asterisk are very tolerant and even favor adolescent male homosexuality.

This does not seem to affect the occurrence of homosexual orientation in adulthood. (Diamond, 1993).

Furthermore, there is no difference in Western societies between the frequency of homosexuality among adults who spent their youth in unisex schools (boys and girls being educated in totally separate locations) or in mixed-sex schools, although it is well known that voluntary homosexual relations occur more frequently in a unisex education environment. If the early life experiences theory had some support, we should expect a higher incidence of homosexuality among adults raised in single-sex schools, which is absolutely not the case (Wellings et al., 1994).

It should be noted that the percentage of adult gay men is remarkably constant in all human societies despite significant differences in the ease with which this orientation is openly accepted. An analysis published by Milton Diamond in 1993 indicated percentages fairly stable between 2 and 8% in societies as diverse as Great Britain, the Netherlands, and the United States. In addition, Diamond did not find any obvious relationship between the attitude of the society vis-à-vis homosexuality and its incidence (see Table 2.1) (Diamond, 1993). The percentage of homosexual men is no higher in very tolerant societies such as the Philippines and Thailand than in societies where it is more difficult to live with a homosexual orientation (Europe, United States). These comparisons across different cultures provide percentages of homosexuality comparable to those reported in the first systematic study of its kind, published by Kinsey (less than 5–10% of men strictly or almost exclusively homosexual in the United States at the time) (Kinsey et al., 1948). These estimates are also confirmed by more recent studies: Mosher and colleagues reported in 2005 that 2 to 3% of men would be preferentially or exclusively homosexual, while the attitude of society vis-à-vis homosexuality has become considerably more lenient (Mosher et al., 2005). This may be anecdotal, but it is intriguing to note that this percentage is in the same order of magnitude as what has been reported for homosexual rams (see Chapter 4). One might therefore wonder whether this percentage might reflect a fairly deterministic mechanism that acts in both animals and humans and is thus more likely biological in nature than environmental.

PSYCHOANALYTIC THEORIES

On the basis of his psychoanalytic practice, Sigmund Freud developed a theory of homosexuality stating that the dynamics of child–parent relationships ultimately determine the sexual orientation of adults. For example, a dominant and possessive mother and/or a distant or absent father might foster a boy developing a homosexual orientation by disrupting the resolution of the Oedipal phase of psychosexual development.

These Freudian and post-Freudian theories were popular for about a half a century, but in recent decades many studies have challenged their scientific validity and even suggested various forms of scientific fraud (from pure lie to partial concealment of results) from Freud himself, and the Oedipal theory has been thoroughly discredited for over two decades now on this basis alone, not to mention that psychoanalysis in general has been described as a nonscientific theory because it is not falsifiable or refutable (Karl Popper sense). It has a reasonable internal consistency but has systematically refused to consider observations going against the theory (Van Rillaer, 1980; Bénesteau, 2002; Dufresne, 2007; Onfray, 2010). In American and British scientific circles, it is now largely ignored, but it must be dealt with here because of its persistence in the culture, since the beliefs of the general public understandably lag behind science's advance.

While some observations seem to support psychoanalytic theory, keep in mind that "correlation is not causation." Thus, while retrospective studies have shown that homosexual men tend to describe their relationship with their mother as closer than the average and with their father as distant and even hostile (Bell et al., 1981; Freund & Blanchard, 1983), it may be that parental attitudes of indifference or hostility toward a child who is going to become homosexual are induced by the character traits of the child that do not meet the expectations of parents. It is in this context important to note that one of the best predictors of adult homosexuality is the presence during childhood of gender-nonconformism. Children that will become gay adults conform less strictly to gender norms. Boys who will become gay engage in less aggressive play, less typical boys' activities, and enjoy interacting with girls and engage in typically female activities. The reverse is true for girls who will later become lesbians. It is thus quite conceivable that the feminized attitude of a pre-gay boy is by itself responsible for the more distant relationship with the father. If the remote or absent attitude of the father were responsible for homosexuality in boys, one would expect an increased incidence of male homosexuality in children raised by single mothers, a situation encountered quite frequently in Western Europe and the United States during the last 20 to 30 years. However, not a single study has been able to identify such an effect.

THEORIES BASED ON LEARNING DERIVED FROM BEHAVIORISM

Following the discovery of numerous rules governing the acquisition of behaviors by classical conditioning (Pavlovian) and especially by operant or Skinnerian conditioning, Behaviorism attached great importance to the influence of learning in the development of animal and human behavior (Skinner, 1965; Richelle, 1966; Skinner, 1971). No behaviorist or psychologist would now defend the idea that behavior can be entirely innate or entirely acquired. All behaviors are partly innate and partly acquired by learning; the respective contribution of these two causes varies according to the behavior in question.

Various learning theorists have suggested that sexual orientation could be the result of conscious and unconscious learning imposed by parents, educators, and even society in general. However, homosexuality does not appear to be a desired character trait in any Western society, so heterosexual parents and educators would not wish to instill homosexuality in their children or students, and probably are doing all they can to prevent its development. This learning could only be transmitted by parents/teachers against their own will. Furthermore, we now have enough data to analyze the fate of children raised by homosexual parents who, we might imagine, might be at least more tolerant even if they do not encourage the development of a sexual orientation identical to their own. However, the data currently available suggest that children of gay parents are generally heterosexual (Stacey & Biblarz, 2001). Similarly, children born to lesbian mothers who are raised by a couple of lesbians are in general heterosexual. Thus, this behaviorist theory has not received support from studies in the last 30 years. Conscious attempts to change the gender identity and sexual orientation of young children also often end in failure (witness the case of John/Joan also called Bruce/Brenda later in this chapter), and numerous attempts to change sexual orientation of gay adults have all completely failed. These attempts included various forms of behavioral therapy and aversive therapy involving the presentation of erotic or pornographic images to homosexuals in association with the swallowing of an emetic (a compound inducing vomiting) or other aversive stimulation (see LeVay, 1996 for more detail). Medical approaches, as well, attempted to "cure" homosexuality–when it was still considered a disease–by radical approaches such as castration, injection of various hormones, electroconvulsive shocks, and even lobotomy (surgical removal of the frontal lobe). American historian Jonathan Katz counted no less than 36 methods used during a century in North America to deal with homosexuality (Katz, 1976). No reproducible results could ever be achieved by all these mutilations or behavioral therapies.

THEORIES BASED ON "SOCIAL CONSTRUCTIVISM"

Social constructivism refers to a current of contemporary sociology that envisages social reality and social phenomena as being "built," i.e., created, institutionalized, and later turned into traditions. Social constructivism focuses on the description of institutions and actions by asking how they "construct" reality. The scientific facts would themselves be products of the dynamics of institutional structures. According to this perspective, sometimes called relativism, truth itself in scientific knowledge would be related to a particular historical and institutional context, and would have no absolute value.

The constructivist school of thought suggests that the development of sexual orientation as hetero-, homo-, or bisexual would simply be a concept imposed by society and internalized by the individual (Halperin, 1990). Some thinkers have even suggested that gender identity would be built and maintained by social interactions (Kessler & McKenna, 1978). Some aspects of sexual identity would be easily learned and not necessarily directly related to reproduction.

Constructivism has contributed to our understanding of human sexuality in its cultural context, but the relevance of this interpretation of sexual orientation appears to be relatively limited. Although gender role is largely socially determined, as noted at the beginning of the book, sex steroids also clearly have a role in some aspects of gender role, as indicated by studies of girls exposed prenatally to abnormally high concentrations of androgens (the congenital adrenal hyperplasy or CAH syndrome) (see Chapters 6 and 8). The determination of gender role is therefore partly in agreement with an explanation based on constructivism, but this is not the case for two other dimensions of sexuality: orientation and gender identity. When they deviate from the "norm" in cases of homosexuality or transsexuality, these two aspects of personality almost always develop in *opposition* to social demands, the opposite of what we would expect if characteristics developed in response to the needs of the family. This interpretation is also contradicted by the comparisons between societies that show that the incidence of homosexuality is relatively constant in different human societies, whatever their attitude toward it. If homosexuality is a cultural construct, its distribution should vary depending on the attitude of society.

No theories that attribute the development of homosexuality to nonbiological causes have produced convincing data to support their interpretations. If any role of social and educational factors exists, that it so far has escaped a rigorous demonstration strongly suggests that these roles are severely limited.

It should be noted that, conversely, biological mechanisms that can reproducibly induce homosexuality in various animal species have been identified, especially by research in genetics and behavioral endocrinology, research that we will spend the bulk of this book examining. All these studies suggest that human or animal homosexuality is the result of an interaction between genetic and hormonal embryonic factors with probably a fairly minor effect of postnatal social and sexual experiences.

BIOLOGICAL CONSTRAINTS ON LEARNING

Nevertheless, many authors, often under the influence of sociology, psychology, or psychoanalysis, believe that human behavior and gender differences that affect this behavior are largely, if not exclusively, the result of learning and social influences. These statements sometimes claim to be based on findings of modern neurobiology that have demonstrated a remarkable plasticity in the structure and function of the human brain during its development and even in adulthood. However, this is an incomplete understanding of recent results in neurobiology. There is indeed a great plasticity of the brain during its development. The human brain is not fully formed at birth, and only a very small percentage of its neurons are mature and connected. During the first few years of life, the vast majority of the neurons that were present at birth will die; only a small number of them (one in ten by some estimates) will survive and be incorporated into functional circuits. The human brain is thus extremely plastic, and this plasticity is guided in part by learning. The adult brain is thus largely the result of experience gained during development. This does not mean, however, that behavioral predispositions do not exist at birth that will resist the potential influence of learning.

Now that the human genome has been sequenced and to some extent interpreted, we know that it contains only 25,000 to 30,000 genes [sequences of deoxyribonucleic acid (DNA) directing the synthesis of one or several proteins; see Chapter 3]. The amount of information contained in these 25,000 genes is far from sufficient to account for the complexity of the tasks that are performed by a human subject and thus by his or her brain. For example, it is impossible to imagine that the different concepts that we master in adulthood–multiplication tables, to take an extreme example–can be encoded in our genetic material. They must be learned. But learning is limited to some extent by the underlying neural structures, and these clearly depend on our genetic heritage. Learning is limited or even impossible in other species that have different genetic makeup (rats; even chimpanzees) or in human beings suffering from a genetic disease that has changed the development of the brain (e.g., some cases of Down syndrome).

Learning takes place in the presence of very specific biological constraints whose complexity is currently being unraveled. For example, modern linguistics suggests that all human languages tend to use the same sounds to describe the mother and father (mama, papa, baba), the first two words that are often made by young children. Some see this as a relic of linguistic structures that were present in the original language spoken by the first humans. Alternatively, given that one limiting factor for language development in young children is the poor motor coordination of the muscles of the larynx, one can also think that this community of early vocabulary stems, at least in part, from the relative ease with which these sounds are pronounced. Language in humans is entirely cultural and learned, but it could be limited, at least partially, by anatomical and physiological constraints. Alternatively, one might even think that some phonemes of human languages are genetically controlled, even if such a proposal will probably always remain impossible to prove. Learning therefore enhances intrinsic genetic properties and, vice versa, genes constrain and limit the potential for learning.

Depending on the physical, functional, or behavioral trait under study, the relative importance of genes or of environment/education varies in a major way, but this control is almost always based on an interaction between these factors. For some physical traits, the innate is obviously much more important, but the genetic message cannot develop without environmental conditions that permit it. For example, the size of an individual has a strong genetic component (parents of tall children are taller than average), but the genetic potential can only be expressed in the presence of adequate supplies of food and good sanitary conditions. This explains the rapid growth of the average stature of the population in Western Europe during the last century. The average size of males was 5'3" in 1900 and reached 5'9" at the end of the 20th century. Such a difference cannot be the result of genetic evolution in such a short period (100 years, about five generations). It is the result of improved living conditions and especially the health care and diet of young children.

I shall not deny here the importance of cultural, educational, and environmental factors. I accept without any problem the idea expressed by Serge Hefez in his latest book: "Sexism in children is in full swing between two and six years when they face all the stereotypes" (Hefez, 2007). Without a doubt, this differential treatment plays a key role in the genesis of many behavioral differences between men and women. Western society's recent evolution to a state of less clearly defined gender roles is accordingly associated with a partial disappearance of these differences (Guiso et al., 2008; Hyde et al., 2008).

However, I believe that these differences do not develop on a *tabula rasa*. Boys and girls are not identical at birth. The presence of a penis in one sex and a vagina in the other are the signs of a deep hormonal imprinting that determined genital form and also most likely modulated the development of certain aspects of the brain's structure and function. Research on animal models has clearly demonstrated the profound and irreversible role of hormones on embryonic brain development and behavior. The action of sex steroids in humans is clearly highlighted by the presence of large sex differences in genital form and reproductive function (see Chapter 6). The study of the human brain also shows that sex steroid receptors are present at the same locations as in animals. Finally, many clinical observations and correlative studies show the existence in humans of indisputable effects of sex hormones on behavior (see Chapter 7).

There are therefore at least traces of behavioral effects of hormones in humans, and a good part of this book will describe the respective contributions of biological (genetic or hormonal) and environmental factors (education, learning) to the control of human behavior. I mainly focus in this context on differences between men and women. I demonstrate that while society indeed plays an important role in the genesis of sex differences by dramatically expanding preexisting differences, the influence of biological mechanisms can clearly be detected in humans. This is especially the case if we look at two specific aspects of reproductive behavior that display sex differences at their largest magnitude: sexual orientation and gender identity.

As we study the influences of hormones on brain development and other biological factors in this book, there are a couple of key concepts to keep in mind: the evolutionary history of life on earth means that we can find evidence of the causes of human behavior through the study of similar behaviors in other animals, and the role of neurons in initiating and controlling our actions.

THE UNITY OF LIFE

Because single-cell organisms evolved into multicellular animals, vertebrates, mammals, apes, and man, all animals and man have parts of their heritage in common. For example, vertebrates, the large animal group to which we belong— which includes fishes, amphibians, reptiles, birds, and mammals—all have in common the same general organization of the body. All are organized around a dorsal nervous system under which there is a spine and then a ventral digestive system.

Similarly, the brains of all vertebrates are formed the same way and are made of similar parts in humans, monkeys, rats, amphibians, and fish. They also deal with information coming from the outside world and control the expression of emotions and behavior through the same cellular mechanisms. This finding is extremely important for the thesis developed in this book. The study of animal behavior and its mechanisms, therefore, forms a logical basis on which to elaborate explanations of human behavior and thus, probably, of homosexuality.

All living creatures, including humans, have a functional organization based on cascades of biochemical reactions that are identical or very similar. For example, almost all these forms of life (with of course a few exceptions due to adaptations) produce their energy by similar chains of biochemical reactions that "burn" sugars into a compound called ATP (an acronym for adenosine triphosphate) capable of providing energy to all parts of the cell where it is required.

All living organisms also share a common system for encoding the genetic information required to build a complete individual from a single cell. In the case of sexual reproduction, adopted by most sophisticated multicellular animals, including humans, the adult will result from an egg fertilized by a spermatozoa.

Genetic information is encoded in all living creatures on earth by special molecules called nucleic acids that exist in two forms: deoxyribonucleic acid (DNA) and ribonucleic acid (RNA). The structure of DNA and RNA is nearly identical (except for a few details) in all living beings; encoding of the information is based on the same four components (adenine, thymine, guanine, and cytosine) organized in two associated strands: the famous double helix of DNA.

This unity of life enables researchers to extrapolate conclusions from studies on animals and thus to draw conclusions for humans. This is one of the important foundations of biomedical research.

NEURONS GOVERN ALL OUR ACTIONS

Before entering the maze of animal research, which strongly suggests that homosexuality in humans or animals has deep biological bases, I would like to review a few philosophical and scientific concepts that are needed to better understand the implications of the experimental data I discuss.

With the development of the neurosciences, the idea that brain activity is the basis for any mental activity took hold. The mainstream of scientific thought now considers the very complex but highly material brain (rather than some nonphysical cause) to be the initiator and controller of behavior, emotions, and thoughts.

Anatomical analysis of the brains of patients who in their lifetimes had experienced brain injuries (mechanical accident; injury by object penetration or stroke) demonstrated already during the 19th century that deficits not only of the motor systems but also of behavioral and cognitive capacities of the patient could often be correlated with the exact location of the lesion as detected postmortem. This approach enabled, for example, the identification of brain areas that control the production of language in humans, areas that were labeled after the names of their discoverers, Pierre Paul Broca (1824–1880) and Carl Wernicke (1848–1905).

Furthermore, during the 20th century, advances in pharmacology made it possible to treat neurological disorders by administration of drugs that affect specific chemical systems of communication between neural cells. Neurons communicate with each other by chemical messengers called neurotransmitters. Any alteration in the activity of these neurotransmitters has deep repercussions, often very specific, on our behavior. Thus, Parkinson's disease, which is characterized mainly by a loss of motor control, results from the degeneration of a particular type of neurons that communicate through a neurotransmitter called dopamine. The decrease of the communication supported by dopamine is responsible for the motor problems observed in Parkinson's patients. If the patient is administered a drug that corrects dopaminergic signaling, his or her motor disorders are corrected at the same time, clear evidence of their specific chemical origin.

At a more complex behavioral level, it is well established that drugs that affect the transmission of information between neurons by another neurotransmitter, serotonin, have reproducible effects on the mood and general state of well-being of the patient. Several drugs are able to change the transmission by serotonin and accordingly have major effects on mood. Also note that addictive drugs (opium, cocaine, heroin, alcohol, etc.) are actually chemical compounds extracted from plants or prepared by man that modify the activity of specific neurotransmitter systems and consequently the perception of the world and the behavior of consumers (Cooper et al., 1996).

Finally, the most accurate data that now support the notion that the brain controls our behavior as well as our mental activity comes from sophisticated studies performed during the last 10 to 20 years thanks to the development of medical imaging techniques such as positron emission tomography (PET) and functional magnetic resonance imaging (fMRI). These techniques, based on principles of physics too complex to be explained here, allow the researcher or the physician to identify brain areas that display, at some point in time, a high electrical or metabolic activity (Miller, 2008; Op de Beeck et al., 2008). This information is collected in the form of anatomical images on a computer screen. It can be obtained from awake patients who must simply remain motionless with their head placed in the imaging device. It is then possible ask the subject to perform a specific task or produce a specific mental activity (e.g., imagine a sequence of words beginning with the same letter, make mental calculations, pretend to play a specific social role, etc.) and to identify which areas of the brain are active at that time. By combining the progress of these imaging techniques with sophisticated experimental protocols, researchers have been able to locate nerve sites controlling subtle mental activities such as handling specific concepts (numbers, words, etc.) or the expression of emotions (anxiety, disappointment, etc.).

We will see that the brain areas that control sexual behavior of mammals are identified and their functioning is well understood. These brain areas are present in humans and are anatomically and functionally very similar to their counterparts in animals. The understanding of human behavior can thus be based, to some extent, on the results of experiments conducted on various species of mammals and other higher vertebrates.

It should nevertheless be noted that if the brain controls behavior, behavior can conversely have a massive impact on brain function and even brain structure. The human brain remains plastic throughout adulthood and is influenced by the lifestyle of an individual and the behavior he or she expresses. For example, it has been shown that London taxi drivers have a hippocampus (a brain structure specialized in the treatment of spatial memory) that is larger than in control individuals. They apparently "develop" this part of their brain by intensive use. This effect of behavior on brain structure obviously complicates the interpretation of many data. The interpretation of correlations between structure and function in the brain must therefore always be done with caution: the direction of causal relationship, if any, is not necessarily obvious.

EDUCATION DOES NOT DETERMINE SEXUAL ORIENTATION AND SEXUAL IDENTITY

Now we return to the topic examined at the start of this chapter: education. It was long believed, and some still believe, that the sexual identity and sexual orientation of an individual are determined by the education received during early childhood. The newborn baby would be completely neutral; during the early years of life after birth the little boy or girl would become aware of his or her sex. The developing baby would build his sexual identity and, correspondingly, establish the foundation for what would later be his sexual orientation based only on the social interactions he would experience.

Sexologists themselves defended until very recently, and some still defend, the idea that sexual identity is a cognitive concept that develops in young children during the early years of life and is completely dictated by the type of education received. The newborn child is from this point of view seen as a *tabula rasa*, and it would be possible to impose the desired identity by appropriate education (Money & Ehrhardt, 1972) and, conversely, inappropriate education could impose an undesired identity. Based on this belief, it was customary in the medical community to assign a gender more or less arbitrarily to children born with intersex genital structures. Since it is easier to surgically reconstruct female (vaginoplasty) than male (penile reconstruction) genital structures in children born with a penis poorly or not developed, female sex was more frequently assigned to children and it was thought that subjects could deal with this assignment very well.

However, this attitude ignores the results of more than 50 years of biological research that has, in recent decades, accumulated data clearly showing that the young baby is not neutral from the sexual point of view. The genetic material of the embryo has led during the early phases of embryonic life to the development of testes or ovaries. The embryo has consequently been exposed to sexually differentiated concentrations of sex steroids (in particular, high levels of testosterone in male embryos) that have a profound influence on later psychosexual development. Much of the present book will be devoted to discussion of these data.

The notion of a hormonal embryonic imprinting connected in normal physiological conditions to genetic sex that has irreversible consequences on further development and on the sexual identity and sexual orientation is slowly finding its place in general public awareness. Medical doctors, and even sexologists, often largely underestimate its importance, yet many clinical cases clearly highlight the permanent effects of the embryonic hormonal milieu. A typical example of this influence hit the headlines in the late 1990s and made a major contribution to the initiation of a change in interpretation of sexual development that I hope will become widespread. Because of its exemplary character and the historic role it played, this clinical case deserves to be exposed in detail here.

Two Canadian monozygotic twins named Bruce and Brian Reimer, born in the early 1960s, were affected at the age of seven months by phimosis, a benign problem in which the glans penis is stuck in the foreskin. Doctors advised the parents to circumcise the children, but during the operation, the penis of Bruce, one of two boys, was completely destroyed by electrocautery. Local doctors indicated to the parents that the mutilated child would be unable in adulthood to have a normal sex life and would suffer from social maladjustment. The parents, who were obviously devastated by this prediction, consulted Professor John Money at Johns Hopkins University to help them decide how to manage this problem.

Because it was impossible at that time to reconstruct by surgery a penis for the boy, Money advised that Bruce be transformed into a girl and raised as such. Indeed, it was thought at the time that if a child were raised in an unambiguous way as a girl, he would develop into a normal heterosexual woman in adulthood (Money & Ehrhardt, 1972). From that time Bruce was thus called Brenda and was dressed and treated like a girl. At the age of two years, the sex change was completed by a medical intervention. The child was surgically castrated and a rudimentary vagina was constructed from the skin of the scrotum. Brenda/Bruce and her/his brother Brian were raised as a brother and sister and monitored periodically by Professor Money, who for years advised parents on what to do to optimize the feminization of Brenda/Bruce.

In the years that followed, scientific reports and presentations at conferences by Professor Money showed that the sex change was a complete success and that Brenda (Bruce) was developing as a normal girl, apart from the fact that she/he was slightly masculine in terms of playing activity (a feature of gender role). According to Money, Brenda/Bruce was copying her/his activities, including domestic activities, from her/his mother, while her/his brother Brian was imitating his father's activities. Brenda/Bruce chose dolls as a gift and Brian chose cars (LeVay, 1996). This case thus supported the contention that culture has a decisive influence on sexual identity and gender role and denied the importance of genetics and biology on human behavior. Sexologists were convinced and claimed that babies are born neutral from the sexual point of view and if you take them early enough and you'll make girls or boys.

Money then lost contact with the family of Brian and Brenda/Bruce. Several decades later (in the 1990s), biologist and sexologist Milton Diamond (University of Hawaii) and his colleague Keith Sigmundson were able to discover what had happened to Brenda/Bruce during late childhood and puberty (Diamond & Sigmundson, 1997). The child was in fact never socialized as a normal girl and he rebelled early. Brenda/Bruce was refusing to wear feminine clothing, urinated standing up, and felt permanently that there was something wrong.

A "female puberty" was induced by treatment with estrogen, but Brenda/Bruce hated her/his breasts and refused the hormone. At the age of fourteen, he/she insisted on knowing the truth, which his/her parents reluctantly revealed. He/she was relieved to finally understand the root of the conflicting feelings he/she experienced. At the age of 15 years, Brenda/Bruce asked people to call him/her David and he went through additional surgery to recover a masculine identity. He underwent a double mastectomy (surgical removal of breasts) and a phalloplasty (surgical reconstruction of a penis). He was also treated with testosterone. He had always been exclusively attracted to women (sexual orientation in agreement with genetic and hormonal sex during embryonic development, not with sex of education during childhood) and, in adulthood, he married a woman with whom he had male-typical sex with his prosthesis. He also adopted children and from that time on lived a relatively normal life as husband and father. Unfortunately he committed suicide at the age of 38 years, for reasons that remain unknown but probably include the breakdown of his marriage, financial difficulties, and the premature death of his brother Brian. His traumatic childhood experiences may have also contributed to this event.

Bruce/Brenda/David Reimer was given the pseudonym of John/Joan in the work of John Money. Before his death in 2004, however, David wanted to make his life experience public so as to prevent such errors from recurring in the future. His story is told in a book written by John Colapinto, *As Nature Made Him: The Boy That Was Raised as a Girl* (New York, Harper Collins, 2000). This story illustrates the dramatic importance of how our society has dealt and still deals with issues related to sexual identity and sexual orientation while ignoring the power of hormonal influences.

This case suggests a conclusion very different from what was widely accepted by Money and his contemporaries in the 1960s. It provides evidence that human beings are not psycho-socially neutral at birth. In keeping with their legacy as mammals, they have trends and predispositions to react according to a male or female pattern. According to Diamond, sexual identity is influenced by social factors but also by the embryonic hormonal environment. John/Joan had obviously been exposed *in utero* to androgen levels typical of a young boy (his penis was normally formed at birth). In this case, the hormonal factors would have outweighed the social influences in determining identity and gender role.

A similar case of penile ablation has been reported (Bradley et al., 1998). This genetically male (XY) subject accidentally lost his penis at the age of two months and was raised as female from the age of seven months on. In adulthood, contrary to John/Joan, he adopted a female sex identity despite the fact that during childhood he enjoyed stereotypically masculine toys and games (partially masculinized sex role). His sexual orientation was essentially bisexual. He was predominantly but not exclusively attracted by women. The role of education as compared to embryonic hormones was thus apparently more prominent in this case than in the patient studied by John Money, possibly because the sex of rearing (as female) was adopted earlier.

It should also be noted that these cases of penile ablation are not isolated and that the conclusions they lead to are reinforced by the analysis of many other clinical conditions. This is particularly true of males suffering from cloacal exstrophy (Chapter 9), a malformation in which external genitalia do not grow during embryonic development. Although "corrected" surgically and raised as girls, many of these subjects have male characteristics and nearly half of them identified as boys and later men.

3

The Hormonal Control of Sexual Behavior

BEHAVIORAL ENDOCRINOLOGY

In this chapter I present a brief review of a mass of data widely accepted in the scientific world concerning the neuroendocrinology of behavior [for a more detailed discussion, interested readers may refer to Becker and colleagues (2002;) and Nelson (2005)]. Although I present a dense array of technical points, I encourage nonscientists to concentrate on general principles rather than trying to understand every single term. In this context it is less important to know exactly what 17β-estradiol and 5α-dihydrotestosterone are and more important to know what they do.

In this section I describe what is known concerning the endocrine control of copulatory behavior in males and females. The elements of hormonal control of these behaviors need not be the same as those of sexual orientation, but recent research has shown that they frequently do overlap. Since much more research has been done concerning copulatory behavior itself, it is clearly useful to first review this huge corpus of data. I then consider what is known specifically about the control of sexual orientation in animals.

From a reductionist point of view, most behaviors can be considered as a series of muscle contractions triggered by a series of organized nerve impulses. To activate a behavioral pattern, a hormone should thus alter the electrical activity in specific neural circuits. This effect can be achieved in particular by changing the concentration and/or activity of neurotransmitters and/or their receptors. At this level, testosterone, estradiol, and progesterone play decisive roles.

By studying the binding sites (receptors) and the action of these hormones in the brain, we have made progress in understanding the neural mechanisms underlying the expression of sexual behavior. The brain is the primary site of action of hormones in relation to the expression of sexual behavior. The peripheral action of hormones may also influence behavior by other means. First, hormones can change the sensory inputs to the brain. For example, androgens affect ejaculation in male rats by increasing the sensitivity of the penis. Estrogens modulate the olfactory sensitivity of females in many species of mammals, including humans. Sexual behavior in mammals is largely induced by olfactory stimuli (pheromones), and thus this variation in olfactory performance could deeply affect behavior. We will see that these olfactory responses are profoundly altered in rodents whose sexual orientation has been altered by hormonal treatments and that remnants of these mechanisms seem to be present in humans.

Second, hormones may influence the development of effector organs such as the muscles that control the syrinx, which is the specialized structure that produces vocalizations in birds. A similar effect exists in humans: testosterone reduces the frequency of the voice in man (makes it deeper) by acting on the structure and muscles of the larynx, and the tone of the voice can be a significant variable in sexual attractiveness.

Finally, hormones can change the social signals provided by external superficial structures. For example, testosterone induces the growth of secondary sexual structures such as the crest of roosters and the antlers of male deer, and these structures in turn modify the interaction of the male with the females of his species. Similar phenomena exist in humans: the secondary sexual structures (beard, body hair, and musculature in men; breasts and wide hips in women) are under the control of sex steroids, and their value as sexual signals is evident. Therefore, hormone-induced behavior modification does not result only from the action of hormones in the brain.

WHICH HORMONES ARE INVOLVED IN THE CONTROL OF SEXUAL BEHAVIOR?

In 1849, Berthold showed that castration of young chicks produces subjects devoid of adult male sexual characteristics (comb and wattles) and lacking sexual behavior. The reimplantation of the testes in these castrated males, however, restored the appearance and behavior of the male (Berthold, 1849). The testicular secretion responsible for these physical and behavioral effects was identified in the early 20th century as testosterone.

As already mentioned, testosterone, or similar androgenic compounds, represents the hormonal stimulus that controls male sexual activity in virtually all vertebrates. In females, estrogens and progestagens play a similar role. It is said that steroids activate sexual behavior. They are not by themselves capable of triggering these behaviors, but they greatly increase the probability of their appearance in the presence of adequate stimuli. In adults of most species, these effects are reversible. They appear after a few days of treatment with sex steroids and disappear at the same speed after castration or ovariectomy.

Other hormones secreted by the adrenal glands (corticosteroids), the pituitary gland (oxytocin, vasopressin), or the hypothalamus also play a role clearly identified in the activation of sexual behavior of males and females, but their analysis is not necessary for the understanding of human behavior and sexual orientation, which are the subject of this book. They are not considered here.

MECHANISMS OF ACTION OF SEX STEROIDS

In almost all vertebrates, the physiological and behavioral aspects of reproduction are thus controlled by a class of steroid hormones called sex steroids [as always, with a few exceptions; see especially the work of David Crews at the University of Texas, Austin (Crews & Gartska, 1982; Crews et al., 1984)]. Steroids are compounds resembling lipids (fatlike) that are synthesized from cholesterol. They are produced in specialized endocrine glands, especially the gonads and adrenal glands. Gonads play a dual role in reproduction. On one hand, they produce reproductive cells (sperm or ova), which after fusion will form the young embryo. On the other hand, they also secrete hormones that control sexual behavior, thus allowing the interactions between the sexes and therefore the encounter of the egg and sperm.

Three major classes of sex steroids are involved in the control of reproduction: androgens, estrogens, and progestagens. Among androgens, the best-known example is testosterone, which is primarily secreted by the testicles. Other, less active, androgens are also produced by the adrenals and may in some pathological cases affect sexual differentiation in girls (see Chapter 6). The ovary is the main source of estrogens, a class of steroids, including estradiol. The ovary produces at other times of the ovarian cycle large quantities of progesterone, the progestagen prototype. These steroids are synthesized by a chain of enzymatic reactions that convert cholesterol into pregnenolone, the precursor of all sex steroids, and then sequentially to progesterone, testosterone, and estradiol in the end (Figure 3.1).

Although androgens are traditionally considered to be male hormones and estrogens/progestagens to be female hormones, testosterone can be transformed, in the ovary but also in the brain, into estradiol through the action of

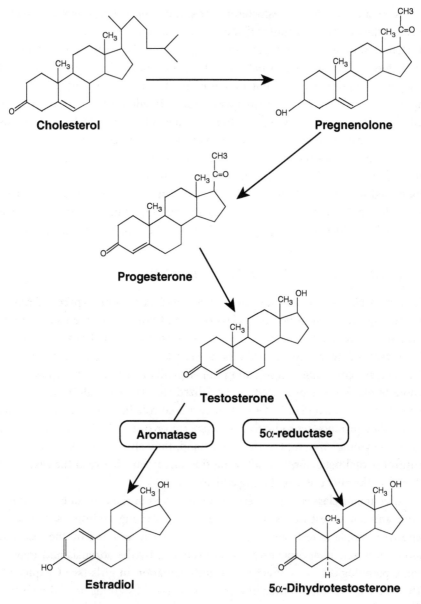

Figure 3.1 Simplified illustration of metabolic pathways for the synthesis of sex steroids from cholesterol.

an enzyme called aromatase. This metabolic conversion plays a crucial role in the control and sexual differentiation of reproductive behavior in mammals and possibly also in humans. Testosterone is also converted in certain target structures into 5α-dihydrotestosterone (by the action of 5α-reductase), and this transformation plays a key role in the action of androgens, particularly in the differentiation of external genital structures (see Chapter 6).

Steroid hormones produce an almost infinite number of physical, functional, and behavioral responses. For example, testosterone is responsible for the growth of the crest of the rooster and the antlers of the deer. It controls the growth of the mammalian penis during puberty and activates male sexual behavior and also aggressiveness. Testosterone or similar androgen synthetic derivatives are used (illegally) by many athletes to increase their athletic performance because androgens also have trophic (nourishing) effects on muscles. Estradiol controls the development of the oviduct in the chicken, as well as in the rat and women. It promotes the development of secondary sexual characteristics such as breasts in women, induces the deposition of yolk (yellow) in the egg of birds and mammals, and activates female sexual receptivity and proceptivity (search for male). More recently it was reported that estradiol also has many other effects outside the field of sexuality. Estradiol and estrogens affect a series of processes of considerable importance in the brain and other organs such as plasticity and neuronal death, the excitability of neurons, the perception of pain (nociception), various complex intellectual processes (memory, attention), and tumor growth in the brain and other organs such as the breast and uterus.

Testosterone, estradiol, and progesterone act on the brain to activate sexual behavior by molecular mechanisms similar to those described for the physical effects at the level of peripheral organs. The sex steroids, as lipophilic compounds (similar to fat), enter freely into their target cells (through the cell membrane) and bind to their specific receptors. The complex formed by the hormone and its receptor acts as transcription factors in the nucleus of these cells to activate or inhibit at the level of DNA the synthesis of new proteins that ultimately change the cells' function. In the brain, these proteins, whose synthesis is modulated by steroids, include receptors (for neurotransmitters, for steroids themselves) and enzymes that modulate the synthesis and degradation (catabolism) of neurotransmitters and receptors.

This type of action, called genomic because it implies a change in the expression of the genome, is by far the best known and probably most important in controlling behavior. The effects it produces are relatively slow (latency of several hours to several days) because the production of new proteins and their incorporation into specific neural circuits is a relatively long process. In addition to this genomic action, steroids, particularly estrogens, are also able to quickly change the physiology of the brain and therefore behavior in a short time, which is hardly consistent with a change in protein synthesis. These effects are induced by interaction with receptors located in the membrane of neurons or by a more or less direct interaction with chains of chemical signaling within neurons. The mechanisms involved remain poorly understood and are currently the subject of a lot of research, namely in our laboratory (see, for example, McEwen & Alves, 1999; Balthazart & Ball, 2006; Cornil et al., 2006; Taziaux et al., 2007; Balthazart et al., 2009; Vasudevan & Pfaff, 2008; Micevych & Dominguez, 2009). I shall not discuss them in this volume, but it is neverthe-less important to bear in mind that steroids are probably able to produce rapid effects on behavior with latencies of about a minute or even a second.

BINDING SITES AND ACTIVITY OF SEX STEROIDS IN THE BRAIN

The anatomical distribution in the brain of sites of action of sex steroids is remark-ably consistent in all vertebrates, including humans. The sites are characterized by neurons expressing specific receptors for these steroids. The receptors are located primarily in the preoptic area, in some parts of the hypothalamus, and in the telencephalon/cerebrum in the structures that are part of the limbic system, such as the amygdala and bed nucleus of the stria terminalis (see Figure 3.2).

Only part of these receptors are involved in the activation of sexual behavior. They were identified by analyzing the behavior of animals that either had been subjected to lesions of small discrete regions of the brain or had been castrated and had received an implant of steroid in a specific brain nucleus. In general the medial part of the preoptic area and ventro-medial nucleus of the hypothala-mus are sites of action of steroids necessary and sufficient to activate male and female sexual behavior, respectively. Implantation of crystals of testosterone in the medial preoptic area of a castrated male is sufficient to restore sexual activity in all species of birds and mammals that were studied (Balthazart & Ball, 2007).

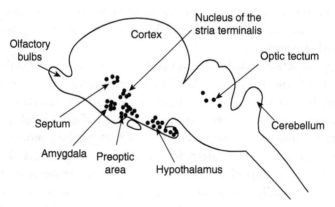

Figure 3.2 Schematic representation of the binding sites of sex steroids in the brain of vertebrates (according to Morrell & Pfaff, 1978).

In females, estradiol and progesterone induce behaviors associated with sexual receptivity by acting in the ventro-medial hypothalamus and in a more caudal part in the posterior mesencephalon (the mesencephalic ventral tegmental area). The action of testosterone in various parts of the limbic system such as the nucleus of the stria terminalis and the amygdala is also important for the activation of male sexual behavior. I shall return to this issue in the discussion of the physical differences of small areas of the brain that are associated with male homosexuality and transsexuality.

CELLULAR MECHANISMS OF ACTION OF STEROID HORMONES

Studies in rats have provided most of the available data on the neurobiological bases of male sexual behavior, but these data seem broadly generalizable to most vertebrate species. The action of testosterone in the medial preoptic area is necessary and sufficient to activate all aspects of sexual behavior in castrated males. Androgens, by binding to their receptors, alter the transcription of specific genes that encode proteins such as neurotransmitter receptors (e.g., for dopamine, norepinephrine) or enzymes that ensure the synthesis or catabolism of these neurotransmitters. These modifications of genomic transcription result in changes in the activity of many neurotransmitters such as dopamine, norepinephrine, and serotonin, which play a key role in the activation of male behavior. Steroids also affect the concentration and release of the specific neuropeptides vasopressin/vasotocin, neuropeptide Y, or gonadoliberin (GnRH) in specific brain structures (Figure 3.3).

Sexual activity of females in many species is limited to a period of a few days (estrus) related to a specific endocrine state. Hormonal determinants of female behavior differ according to species. In rats, for example, the sexual receptivity associated with estrus is induced by elevated circulating levels of estrogen, for about two days, followed by a peak of progesterone. Ovariectomy removes all aspects of female sexual behavior, but behaviors can be reactivated in ovariectomized females by hormonal treatment that mimics the hormonal sequence of events (sequential treatment with estrogen and progesterone) normally observed during the ovarian cycle. In other species (e.g., prairie vole, ferret), estrogens alone are fully able to activate sexual receptivity in ovariectomized females. Just as testosterone does in the male, estradiol, associated or not to progesterone, activates behavior by acting in specific regions of the brain to modify the activity of many neurotransmitters and neuropeptides by changing either their synthesis/degradation or the concentration of their receptors.

Many details remain to be researched before we fully understand these processes. However, we can say that in rats and in most other animal models, the complex neurochemical mechanisms described above are responsible for the

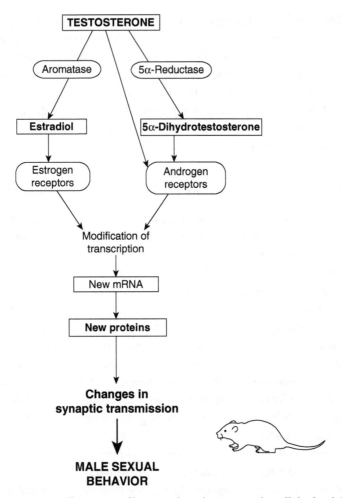

Figure 3.3 Schematic illustration of hormonal mechanisms at the cellular level that activate the expression of male sexual behavior in vertebrates.

activation of sexual behavior. Based on the continuity of evolutionary and brain physiology between man and animals, we may think that this conclusion also applies, at least in part, to humans. Given the moral impossibility of performing direct experiments in humans, this conclusion is obviously supported by less direct arguments (e.g., the analysis of clinical cases). Although it is also clear that the behavioral and cognitive development of humans is far more complex than that of animals, and neurotransmission mechanisms that underlie behavior are also of great complexity, there is no logical reason to believe that qualitatively different phenomena are brought into play at the human level.

INTRACELLULAR METABOLISM OF STEROIDS

After they have entered their target cells in the brain but before binding to their receptors, some steroids, particularly testosterone, are submitted to important metabolic changes. Two enzymes (aromatase and 5α-reductase) catalyze the conversion of testosterone into behaviorally active metabolites, namely 17β-estradiol and 5α-dihydrotestosterone (DHT: see Figure 3.1), respectively. Depending on the species, 17β-estradiol and DHT, alone or in synergy, reproduce most, if not all behavioral effects of testosterone. The male copulatory behavior may, for example, be activated by DHT alone in rabbits or in guinea pigs, and by estradiol-17β alone in rats and Japanese quail. In rats, estradiol-17β, a hormone classically regarded as "female," is responsible for the activation of male copulatory behavior if we look at the level of neurons where this activation takes place. This conclusion could also be applicable, at least in part, to man (Bagatell et al., 1994; Carani et al., 1999; Carani et al., 2005). In most species, the two metabolites of testosterone, however, act synergistically and a more intense response is observed after simultaneous treatment by DHT and 17β-estradiol. The importance of the relative role of estrogen (17β-estradiol) and androgen (DHT) metabolites from testosterone varies greatly from species to species, and experimental data are partially lacking in humans, thus preventing an entirely accurate assessment of its relative importance.

The activity of enzymes that metabolize testosterone varies in different regions of the brain in specific ways depending on factors such as gender, age, season, or hormonal status of the subjects. This produces a local variation of the quantity of metabolites' behavioral assets, which provides a mechanism to precisely modulate the action of steroids on behavior.

HORMONES AND SEXUAL MOTIVATION

Sexual behavior is divided by ethologists into two distinct components: an appetitive component that includes all behaviors to allow the encounter of the two sexes (partner search, approach, sexual displays) and a consummatory aspect (performance) represented by the act of mating itself (Marler & Hamilton, 1966; Everitt, 1995; Balthazart et al., 2009). The majority of studies on the neurobiology of sexual behavior have been devoted to the analysis of the consummatory aspects, but a substantial amount of work has also been devoted to the appetitive component, also called anticipatory phase or sexual motivation. The male sexual motivation can be measured indirectly in animals by quantifying the time latency between the introduction of a female in the cage of a male and his first sexual reaction, the number and persistence of pursuits of the female in an experimental cage with several compartments, or the willingness to endure an aversive stimulus (electrified grid) or the activity in an operant conditioning procedure to access the female.

It is interesting to note that hormonal stimuli that activate sexual motivation appear identical to those involved in controlling performance. This can be understood from a evolutionary point of view: for the reproduction of the species, it is essential that the two phases of behavior take place in sequence, and it is therefore logical that the evolution has selected identical or at least very similar mechanisms to control the two phases of behavior. Depending on the species, the DHT and/or 17β-estradiol formed by aromatization of testosterone in the preoptic area and hypothalamus stimulate full appetitive sexual behavior in castrated males. However, distinct regions of the preoptic area seem to control the appetitive and consummatory aspects of sexual behavior in male quail, and studies in rats indicate a double dissociation between the neuroanatomical sites responsible for two aspects of behavior (Everitt, 1990; 1995). Indeed, it appears that in rats, lesions of the medial preoptic area suppress copulatory behavior but leave intact sexual motivation as measured by the pressure of a lever finally giving access to a sexually receptive female in an operant conditioning cage. Furthermore, lesions of the amygdala drastically reduce sexual motivation without affecting performance. The interpretation of these data is complex, however, and there are still many questions concerning the sites involved in the nervous control of various components of sexual behavior. These sites appear to be similar, but differences might also exist (Balthazart & Ball, 2007). In contrast, it seems that the same steroids activate the two phases of sexual behavior.

SEX DETERMINATION AND SEXUAL DIFFERENTIATION

DNA during cell division is concentrated in the nucleus to form small rods called chromosomes, which are visible under a microscope. There are 23 pairs in humans. In 22 of them, the two chromosomes are identical and each contains a copy of any genetic information inherited in part from the mother and partly from the father. The 23rd pair is formed in men (males) from two different chromosomes, one called X and a much shorter one called Y. Women (females) have two X chromosomes. These chromosomes separate during the cell division that precedes the formation of sperm and egg cells (meiosis). All eggs obviously contain an X chromosome, but sperm cells have either an X or a Y. Depending on whether the egg is fertilized by an X or Y sperm, the embryo formed–and later the individual–will be respectively a woman (XX) or man (XY). This system of sex determination operates in an identical manner in all mammals that have been studied. Only the total number of chromosomes varies from one species to another.

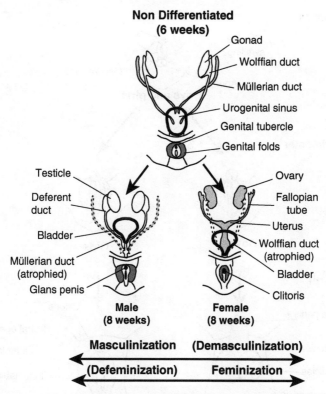

Figure 3.4 Schematic representation of the sexual differentiation process of internal sexual organs in humans. Müllerian and Wolffian ducts are both present in the undifferentiated embryo 6 weeks after conception. Under the influence of hormones produced by the testes, the Müllerian ducts (in gray) regress and Wolffian ducts develop in vas deferens and seminal vesicles. In the absence of testosterone, Wolffian ducts (white) regress and Müllerian ducts develop in the fallopian tubes and uterus.

In early embryonic development, there is no visible difference between the genital structures, internal or external, in the male and female embryos. It is said that the sexual phenotype is undifferentiated (see Figures 3.4, 3.5). The embryonic tissue that will form the embryonic gonad, a generic term referring to the testicles and ovaries, is identical for both sexes, and the genital tract contains both types of ducts: the Müllerian ducts (sketches for future female genital tract) and the Wolffian ducts (drafts of the male genital tract).

From this undifferentiated stage, sexual differentiation proceeds in two steps. The DNA of the Y chromosome contains a gene (SRY, for sex-determining region of the Y chromosome) that induces the synthesis of a protein called TDF (testis-determining factor). This protein alone determines the formation of a male embryo.

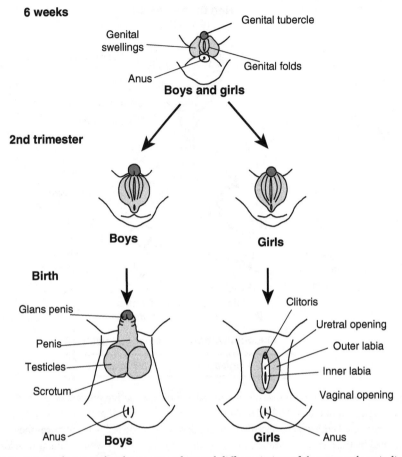

Figure 3.5 Embryonic development and sexual differentiation of the external genitalia in humans. A single genital outline is present at six weeks after conception. Under the influence of testicular testosterone and its metabolite, 5α-dihydrotestosterone, the genital folds fuse to form the scrotum and the genital tubercle develops in the penis. Without these hormones, genital folds form the labia of the vulva and genital tubercle forms the clitoris.

In a first step during the early embryonic development, the SRY gene is activated and its transient expression in the gonads results in the synthesis of TDF protein in specific cells that are the future Sertoli cells. This TDF protein stimulates, directly or indirectly, the expression of many genes (organizers or architect genes) that lead to the differentiation of the undifferentiated gonad into testis. There is no SRY gene on chromosome X and, therefore, in the absence of the protein TDF, the primordial gonadal tissue will not produce a testis. In humans, differentiation of the female ovaries, however, is a complex process that is still not fully understood and involves additional control factors.

During the second stage, specialized cells of the differentiated testis will begin to secrete two chemical messengers, the testicular hormones, which will spread in the whole body to organize it into a male individual (man). The interstitial cells (Leydig cells) secrete testosterone, which determines the genitals' form [fusion of the lips (labia) of the vulva to form a scrotum and development of the genital tubercle to form a penis (see Fig. 3.5)] and maintenance of Wolffian ducts (which form the epididymis, the vas deferens, and seminal vesicles). Testosterone is also implicated in the development and organization in a male direction of all physical and behavioral characters that are sexually differentiated. Another type of testicular cell (Sertoli cells) in parallel will produce anti-Müllerian hormone, which induces the regression of the Müllerian ducts. The establishment of the male sex phenotype is therefore under the action of two testicular hormones, testosterone and anti-Müllerian hormone.

In females, the gonads become ovaries. The absence of testicular hormones is responsible for the persistence of the Müllerian ducts, disappearance of the Wolffian ducts, and development of external female genitalia (labia majora and minora, clitoris, feminization of the genitalia). The development of the female phenotype is for the most part spontaneous. It occurs in the absence of SRY and hence in the absence of testosterone and anti-Müllerian hormone. The female sex is considered the "default" sex, since it develops in the absence of a specific genetic or hormonal influence.

In summary, sexual differentiation takes place in two stages, a first leading from genetic sex to gonadal sex and a second during which the gonadal sex induces, by hormonal influences, the phenotypic sex differences. At birth, the sexual phenotype is visible in many mammals, including humans. The sexual organs are differentiated, but these organs are not functional. It is only at puberty that the hormones (testosterone in males and estradiol/progesterone in the females), secreted by the gonads in increasing quantities, will take control of the reproductive function of typical adult. These hormones then control the final maturation of the reproductive tract, the appearance of secondary sexual characteristics, and sexual behavior.

BEHAVIORAL SEX DIFFERENCES AND ORGANIZATIONAL EFFECTS OF STEROIDS DURING DEVELOPMENT

Many behaviors in animals and humans are sexually differentiated and are produced preferentially or exclusively by one sex. These behavioral differences partly result from the presence of various hormones in adult males and females (testosterone and estradiol/progesterone, respectively). However, in many species, the activation of male copulatory behavior is dependent at the cellular level on the action of estradiol (a hormone characteristic of females), which is produced by aromatization of testosterone in the brain. It is not the type of hormone that determines the type of behavior that is produced, but rather the neural substrate on which this hormone acts, with the nature of the neural substrates depending on the sex of the subject. Estrogens are often unable to activate behavior typical of females (e.g., responsiveness) in males, and testosterone does not activate mounting behavior in females even after its conversion into estradiol.

We now know that these sexually differentiated behavioral responses to steroids are the result of early actions of these steroids and that during ontogeny the brain differentiates into a male or female brain. These differentiating effects occur during the embryonic period or just after birth and are completely irreversible. In mammals, the early exposure to testosterone produces a male phenotype: the behavioral characteristics of the male are strengthened (masculinization) and the ability of males to show behavior typical of females is reduced or lost (defeminization). The female phenotype apparently develops in the absence of hormone (or in the presence of very low levels of estrogen). In summary, the female phenotype develops spontaneously in the relative absence of hormones but testosterone is required to impose masculinity. The differentiation process that takes place spontaneously during the early development of animals can be reproduced at will by experimental manipulation of circulating concentrations of steroids in embryos or newborn animals (Figure 3.6).

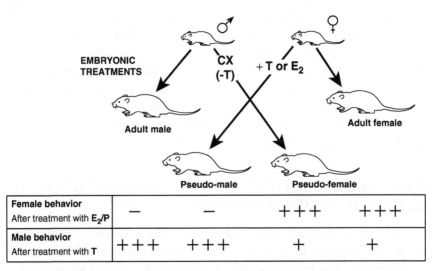

Female behavior After treatment with E$_2$/P	–	–	+++	+++
Male behavior After treatment with T	+++	+++	+	+

Figure 3.6 Schematic representation of the hormonal processes during ontogenesis that induce sexual differentiation of brain and behavior. CX: castration; T: testosterone; E2: estradiol; P: progesterone. + + + Behavior regularly expressed; + rare behavior; – behavior absent.

Thus, the injection of testosterone in an embryonic female rat produces a profound masculinization of sexual behavior. This genetic female is capable as an adult of responding to injections of testosterone by producing the full range of sexual behaviors typical of males. Conversely, if a newborn male is castrated at birth, his behavior will not be fully masculinized and he will be unable in adulthood to achieve the behaviors typical of his sex with high frequency. Correlatively, his sexual behavior is not defeminized: he is capable of producing the female posture of sexual receptivity (lordosis) in response to a sequential treatment with estradiol and progesterone. Thus, the behavioral phenotype of rats can be completely reversed by early hormonal manipulation. One can produce individuals who will, in adulthood, exhibit the behavioral characteristics of males or females regardless of the genetic sex of individuals (Goy & McEwen, 1980).

As shown in Figure 3.6, prenatal injection of testosterone (but also of estradiol) masculinizes sexual behavior in female rats. This observation stems from the fact that testosterone masculinizes behavior during ontogeny largely through its conversion into estradiol (by aromatization in the brain). This notion is confirmed by the finding that if a genetic male, whose embryonic testis produces large quantities of testosterone, is injected during the last week of uterine life and the first week of postnatal life with an aromatase inhibitor, that is, a compound that pharmacologically blocks the conversion of testosterone to estradiol, sexual behavior will not be fully masculinized. It therefore appears that the effects of testosterone in rats are produced at the cellular level by estradiol derived from aromatization, both during ontogeny (masculinization of behavior) and during adulthood (activation of sexual behavior mature). In the next two paragraph, I discuss two other aspects of the mechanisms of hormonal control of sexual differentiation of behavior that also have a significant impact on the interpretation of homosexual behavior and its possible hormonal origin.

It is very important to note that the changes of behavioral sex produced by testosterone or estradiol occur only during a limited and well-defined period of development of the animal. This period is called the **critical period** and corresponds to a stage of brain development during which the brain is still very plastic and can therefore be changed by exposure to sex steroids. In rats, a species in which the young are born at an early stage of development (they are naked, blind, do not regulate their body temperature, and are unable to move by themselves), this period is essentially the last week of embryonic life and the first week of postnatal life. In other species, such as the guinea pig, where the young are more developed at birth, this period of brain development takes place entirely during embryonic life and, therefore, the critical period of sexual differentiation is entirely prenatal.

It is also important to note that all these organizing effects of steroids are completely *irreversible*. If testosterone or estradiol are present during the critical period and have the opportunity to masculinize and/or defeminize sexual behavior, these effects will be present during the entire life of the animal. A female who has been masculinized and defeminized by early exposure to testosterone (or estradiol) is unable during her whole life to present the behavior of lordosis in response to an appropriate treatment by estradiol and progesterone in adulthood. Correlatively, this masculinized female responds to treatment with testosterone in adulthood by showing copulatory behavior typical of the male. This reaction, normally characteristic of the male, remains masculinized in the female throughout her life. Conversely, a male castrated immediately after birth can display lordosis behavior for all his life but never responds in adulthood to treatment with testosterone. Contrary to the *activating* effects of steroids, which are fully reversible and are seen only during the period of exposure to hormones, the *organizing* effects are permanent and last for the entire life of the animal from the time they were induced during early life.

The mechanisms of hormonal control of sexual differentiation of behavior have now been identified in many species of mammals and birds and thus appear to be general, although there are fine differences in the mechanisms involved. Thus, the relative importance of the process of masculinization and defeminization varies from one species to another. For example, sexual differentiation of male rats involves an almost complete defeminization linked to a limited behavioral masculinization, whereas in rhesus monkeys there is rather a marked masculinization of behavior that is not associated with an important process of defeminization.

More subtle differences in exposure to hormones during development can also influence the differentiation of behavior. A female rat embryo placed between two males in the uterus will be exposed to concentrations of steroids slightly higher and, when an adult, will show higher levels of male-typical behavior than will control females.

Defeminization and masculinization of male mammals are induced by testicular androgens; however, it is not testosterone itself that differentiates the brain but its metabolite produced by aromatization in the brain, estradiol. The ovaries of pregnant females produce high amounts of estradiol, which passes the placental barrier easily. One might therefore wonder why the maternal estrogen does not also masculinize female embryos. Plasma from rat embryos contains a protein secreted by the liver, alpha-fetoprotein (AFP), which binds with high affinity to estrogens and prevents them from entering the brain (Bakker et al., 2006). This is why all embryos are not masculinized and defeminized by maternal estrogens. However, AFP does not bind to testosterone, which, after being secreted by the testes, can reach the male brain where it exerts its effects after being aromatized to estradiol locally.

Some species, such as primates, do not appear to have discernible levels of circulating AFP. The relative importance of the aromatization of testosterone in the brain to sexual differentiation is also variable from one species to another, and, in monkeys, for example, androgens themselves seem more important than estrogens. Extrapolation to humans of the mechanisms described on the basis of studies in animals should thus be made with due caution and still requires verifications that must be based on clinical or epidemiological studies. However, the main principles of control of sexual differentiation deducted from animal studies appear to be applicable to humans (see Chapter 6). Differences between species lie in the details.

THE SEXUALLY DIMORPHIC NUCLEUS OF THE PREOPTIC AREA, AND OTHER SEXUALLY DIFFERENTIATED NEURAL STRUCTURES

When the process of sexual differentiation of reproductive behavior was first identified in the late 1950s, it was thought that the brains of males and females were physically identical. Researchers naturally assumed that, during perinatal life, hormones defeminized/masculinized reproductive behavior by changing specific aspects of the physiology of the brain irreversibly (such as the functioning of specific neurotransmitter systems), but these physiological changes were not reflected in the neuronal structure of affected animals.

In the decade that followed, however, a few researchers analyzed the brains of males and females in more detail with the hope of finding physical differences between sexes. In 1969 Günter Dörner demonstrated that a specific part (the nucleolus) of the nucleus of neurons in an area of the hypothalamus (the ventro-median hypothalamus, which controls the expression of female sexual behavior) is larger in female rats than in male rats (Dörner & Staudt, 1969). A few years later, Raisman and Field demonstrated via electron microscopy that synapses in the ventro-medial hypothalamus are different in males and females and, most important, that this sexual difference develops under the action of testosterone during perinatal life (Raisman & Field, 1971). The treatment of young female rats with testosterone induced synaptic connections of the male type. This correlation suggested that the change in synaptic connectivity is causally involved in the sexual differentiation of reproductive behavior. The morphological differences known in the early 1970s, however, were details of organization at the subcellular level, and it was then still believed, on a more macroscopic level, that the brain of males was identical to that of females.

A discovery made in canaries altered that view. In the canary, as in many other birds of the group called passerines or songbirds, males are characterized by the abundant expression of song during the reproduction period, whereas singing is generally absent or much more discrete in females. In the early 1970s, Fernando Nottebohm and his colleagues at the Rockefeller University in New York identified the neural circuits that control song, and two years later Fernando Nottebohm and Art Arnold discovered that several components of this neural circuit are affected by a major physical sex difference (Nottebohm & Arnold, 1976). In particular, three groups of neurons of the telencephalon—HVC (formerly known as the high vocal center), RA (the robust nucleus of the arcopallium), and area X of the medial striatum—have a volume two to five times larger in males than in females, depending on the species considered. The difference in size is so great that it can be seen with the naked eye in a brain section stained by appropriate methods.

The discovery of a large neuroanatomical sex difference in songbirds led various researchers to reconsider the idea that such differences did not exist in mammals. In particular, the group of Professor Roger Gorski (University of California at Los Angeles) re-analyzed the structure of the preoptic area in male and female rats. He discovered the existence of a sexually dimorphic nucleus (SDN) in the preoptic area of this species (Gorski et al., 1978). This difference is also very important: the SDN of the male rat is five times larger than the SDN of females, and this difference may also be seen with the naked eye on a brain section prepared for microscopic examination (see Figure 3.7).

The location of this nucleus in the middle of the preoptic area—which is, remember, the area of the brain involved in a privileged way in the activation by

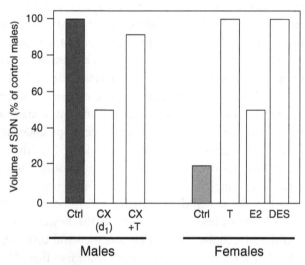

Figure 3.7 In rats, the volume of the sexually dimorphic nucleus (SDN) of the preopic area is about five times larger in males than in females—a difference induced by steroids during the perinatal life. Castration (CX) during the first day after birth (d1) reduces nucleus size in males, and this may be offset by treatment with testosterone (T). Perinatal treatment of females with testosterone, estradiol (E2), or a synthetic estrogen (DES) increases the volume of this nucleus, but these organizing effects will only be observed later in adulthood (according to Gorski, 1984).

testosterone of male sexual behavior—strongly suggests that the nucleus plays a key role in controlling the behavior. Many experiments have been conducted to test this idea and have so far obtained only a partially positive answer. It was shown that lesions in the preoptic area covering all or part of the SDN inhibit the expression of male copulatory behavior but that more discrete lesions localized specifically at the SDN are usually without effect. It seems that the SDN and the preoptic area that surrounds it are involved in the expression of male sexual behavior but the specific lesion of SDN is generally insufficient to inhibit behavior.

The analysis of the hormonal mechanisms that control the volume of the rat SDN, however, provides additional suggestions of a causal relationship between the size of the nucleus and behavioral activity. The size of the male rat SDN does not depend on the hormonal status of animals in adulthood but rather is determined by the endocrine environment experienced by the animal during the last week of embryonic life and the first week of postnatal life. Thus the injection of testosterone in young females during this critical period produces adult females displaying a size of the SDN identical to that of a male (which is five times greater than in untreated females). Conversely, if a small male rat is castrated at birth, the size of his SDN in adulthood is significantly lower than that of a typical male (about half). However, the castrated rat's SDN is larger than in a female because, as explained above, the differentiation of the SDN is induced by testosterone in the last week of prenatal life and in the first postnatal weeks. Castration at birth interrupts a process that is already under way, and the size of the SDN is already greater than in a female who has never been exposed to testosterone (see Figure 3.7). Once the nucleus size is determined at the end of the first week of postnatal life, it is fixed for life; and like the type of sexual behavior (male or female), this feature cannot be changed by hormone treatments in adulthood.

It should be noted that the "masculinization" of the volume of SDN by perinatal actions of testosterone is induced at the cellular level by estrogens produced in the brain by aromatization of testosterone. This conclusion is amply demonstrated by the finding that injection of estrogen increases the SDN volume in the same way as testosterone (if the injected dose is sufficient to saturate the binding capacity of alpha-fetoprotein, or if a specific estrogen such as diethylstilbestrol, DES, which does not bind to alpha-fetoprotein, is used). Furthermore, injection of an aromatase inhibitor blocks the effects of testosterone on masculinization of the volume of SDN. These experimental arguments, and others not described here, therefore demonstrate with confidence, in rats at least, that the masculinization of the SDN induced by testosterone is produced in the brain by estrogens that are derived by aromatization.

Following this discovery of the SDN in rats by Roger Gorski and his staff, many similar sexually dimorphic structures have been discovered in the preoptic area of many other species of mammals, including humans (see Chapter 4), birds, reptiles, and amphibians. These dimorphic structures of the preoptic area are apparently not homologous in different species and are not necessarily controlled by the same hormonal mechanisms. The larger size in males of the preoptic SDN is indeed, in some species such as adult Japanese quail, the result of the presence of a higher concentration of testosterone in males than in females. In technical terms, this difference is linked to a different activation in adulthood by steroids rather than to a differential organization during early life. It seems that in most mammals studied, the sexual dimorphism in the size of the SDN of the preoptic area is the result of a differentiation by sex hormones during early life, either embryonic or immediately postnatal.

Finally, following this identification of an SDN in the preoptic area in many species, neuroanatomists have analyzed the possible existence of physical differences between other parts of the brains of males and females. They have identified a variety of structures that are either larger in males than in females (nucleus of the stria terminalis in rats) or in females than in males (ventromedial nucleus of the hypothalamus). I return to this topic in more detail when analyzing the physical differences between the brains of men and women (Chapter 6).

4

Biological Determinism of Sexual Orientation in Animals

All studies of hormonal control of behavior and sex differences described in the previous chapter deal exclusively with the mechanisms that determine the type of behavior performed by the animal at a given time. This research, which is focused on determining the origins of sex differences affecting behavioral activity in the stricter sense, is of limited usefulness to explain human behavior. The behavioral differences between men and women are indeed numerous and include sexual orientation, which is the subject of this book. However, it is clear that these differences do not concern the kind of sexual behaviors produced by men and women. There is no stereotypical position adopted by men and women in sexual relationships. Sexual relations between men and women occur in a variety of positions and without systematic differences behavior patterns. These positions vary from one moment to another and from one culture to another. They are largely determined by cultural influences, but are neither stereotypical nor probably controlled by specific biological or hormonal mechanisms. Animal research on the analysis of mechanisms of hormonal controls of motor patterns differentially expressed by males and females therefore proposes at best analogous models for differences that affect the sexual behavior and sexual orientation of humans.

Unlike other aspects of human sexuality that have no equivalent in the animal (e.g., gender role or sexual identity, see Chapter 5), sexual orientation can be

easily studied in animals. The test animal can be offered a choice between
a male or female sexual partner, and the observer can record toward which
of these partners the test animal orients its sexual behavior. This type of research
is not as developed as the research on sexual behavior in the stricter sense, and
it was started more recently. However, two important principles are already
firmly established: (1) that the sexual orientation of reproductive behavior is
controlled, both in adulthood and during its development from conception
through maturation, by the same hormones that control sexual behavior, and
(2) that these hormones act in the same brain regions to activate sexual behavior and determine its orientation. I summarize these data in the following
pages as they establish the theoretical context from which I propose thereafter
an explanatory model of human homosexuality based on early (embryonic)
and irreversible effects of sex steroids.

SEXUAL ORIENTATION IN ANIMALS IS CONTROLLED
BY THE HYPOTHALAMUS

In animals as in humans, sexual orientation is a characteristic of reproductive
behavior that is strongly differentiated between males and females. Most sexual
activity of males is oriented toward females and vice versa. This orientation can
be quantified in standardized experimental conditions in cages with three compartments (see Figure 4.1).

The test animal is placed in the central compartment of the cage and a stimulus male and stimulus female are randomly placed in the left and right compartments. The stimulus subjects are maintained by a harness or another similar
experimental device that prevents their passage into the central cage, while
allowing the test animal to freely visit the three compartments. This experimental procedure was used for a variety of animal species, but the most detailed
data are available for the laboratory rat (*Rattus norvegicus*) and the ferret
(*Mustela putorius*). It was observed, as might be expected, that in such a device
males spend most of their time (often more than 80–90%) in the compartment
containing a sexually receptive female, with whom the male will mate. He will
visit the compartment containing a male for much less time, and in his presence he will exhibit only investigative or aggressive behaviors. A sexually
mature and receptive female will spend most of her time in the compartment
containing a male with whom she will mate even if he is held captive in his
compartment.

The neuroendocrinologists studying behavior showed that the preference
of males or females for the compartment containing a subject of the opposite
sex is controlled by steroid hormones that, in parallel, modulate the expression
of male copulatory behavior and female responsiveness. The castration of the

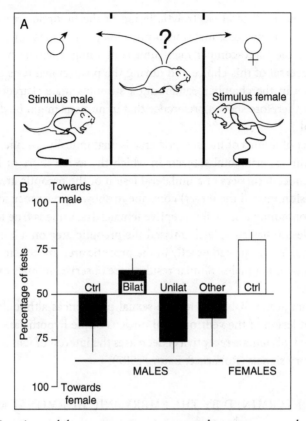

Figure 4.1 Experimental three-compartment cages used to measure sexual orientation in small rodents and in ferrets (A), and effect of lesions of the medial preoptic area on these preferences in the ferret (B). Male control ferrets (Ctrl) visit the compartments containing females for most of the test time and control females preferentially visit the male compartments. Male preferences are reversed following a bilateral lesion (Bilat) of the preoptic area but not by unilateral lesions (unilateral) or lesions of a different site of the brain (Other) (according to Paredes & Baum, 1995).

male or the female ovariectomy eliminates or greatly reduces the preference of the experimental subject for the compartment containing a subject of the opposite sex.

A limited number of studies have also researched which nerve sites underlie the expression of these preferences. Overall these studies show that sexual preferences are controlled in males by the medial preoptic area. The first experiments supporting this conclusion, and probably the most convincing, were obtained in the ferret by Michael Baum and his colleagues at Boston University.

Like the rat, the ferret has a sexually dimorphic nucleus at the level of the medial preoptic area. Its volume is significantly larger in males than in females.

If we carry out a bilateral electrolytic lesion of the preoptic area at the level of this dimorphic nucleus, males who previously spent most of their time in the room of the three-compartment unit containing a female have a nearly complete reversal of this choice and during the postlesional tests spend most of their time in the chamber containing a stimulus male (Paredes & Baum, 1995). They therefore show a preference that in humans might be described as homosexual.

This effect of lesions of the preoptic area is anatomically specific, as demonstrated by the experimental subjects in which the lesion more or less missed the target. Indeed, carriers of a unilateral lesion of the preoptic area (the contralateral lesion missed the target) continue to show a preference for the compartment containing a sexually receptive female. The same is true for males in whom the lesion has completely missed the preoptic area on a bilateral basis. Only bilateral lesions placed exactly in the preoptic area are able to reverse the sexual orientation of males. Similar results were observed in male rats (Paredes et al., 1998).

Fewer data are available for female sexual preferences although one study showed that lesion of the ventromedial nucleus of the hypothalamus (a structure that controls female receptivity) decreases the interest of female ferrets for male olfactory signals (Robarts & Baum, 2007).

... AND DETERMINED BY THE EMBRYONIC HORMONAL MILIEU

The same type of experiment was used to investigate how these sexual preferences develop during ontogenesis. More specifically, the researchers wondered whether hormonal mechanisms identical or at least similar to those that induce the differentiation of sexual behavior (see Chapter 3) control the organization of its orientation. A positive response was given to this question.

We have seen previously that embryonic testosterone is responsible for the masculinization of reproductive behavior in male rats. This effect is produced in neurons by the action of estradiol produced by aromatization of testosterone. Indeed, injection of an aromatase inhibitor during the end of embryonic life or during the first week of postnatal life inhibits masculinization of behavior. It was also demonstrated that the same treatment by an aromatase inhibitor blocks, to a large extent, the development of heterosexual preference in male rats (Bakker et al., 1993a; Bakker et al., 1996b).

When tested in adulthood in a cage with three compartments (similar to that described in the previous section), rats in which aromatase was blocked during the perinatal period spend, unlike normal rats, the majority of their time in the compartment containing another male and largely ignore the compartment containing a sexually receptive female. Moreover, these rats rarely attempt to mate with sexually receptive females that are present and, even more tellingly, allow the male stimulus to mount them. They are thus showing a form of sexual preference that, in humans, would be qualified as homosexuality or at least bisexuality. In addition, these rats have, as adults, a small SDN in the preoptic area (see previous chapter), which is characteristic of the female (Houtsmuller et al., 1994). It therefore appears that absence of estrogen exposure in male rats during the perinatal life has a lasting effect on the sexual preferences of the male in adulthood. These rats are not masculinized and tend to prefer other males to females.

Recent studies confirm this interpretation by showing that the treatment (during the first three weeks of life) of young female rats with estrogen (estradiol benzoate) has the opposite effect. This treatment increases their preference for females, a preference that would be classified as homosexual in women (Figure 4.2) (Henley et al., 2009) (see Henley et al., 2011 for review). These preference tests were conducted at the adult age in ovariectomized females subjected to various hormone treatments (estrogen alone or estrogen plus progesterone) to activate different aspects of sexual behavior. The preference reversal was observed in both hormonal conditions, thus suggesting that "homosexual" preferences induced by perinatal treatment cannot be modified by hormones in adulthood.

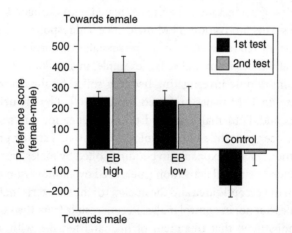

Figure 4.2 Effect of treatment with an estrogen, estradiol benzoate (EB), at high or low dose, during the first three weeks of life on the sexual preferences of female rats. The preference score represents the time spent by the animal in the test chamber containing a female minus the time spent in the chamber containing a male. A negative score indicates a preference for males (usually observed in female controls). A positive score indicates a reversal of this choice (preference for female) following treatment with EB at both doses used (according to Henley et al., 2009).

The brains of "homosexual" male rats described above also respond in an atypical manner to the presentation of olfactory stimuli of a sexual nature. In control animals, the nuclei that process olfactory information in relation to sexual behavior are indeed activated in males by presenting odor typical of females (i.e., the cage bedding soiled by a female's urine), while the female brain is activated by the odor of the male. In contrast, the brain of a control male is not activated by the presentation of a litter soiled by a male, and vice versa. This is very different in male rats treated during the perinatal period with an aromatase inhibitor: their brain is instead highly activated by the odor of other males (Bakker et al., 1996a). This change in early hormonal environment has apparently produced a profound change in what the animal sees as sexually attractive or exciting. We shall see that similar changes in brain activity induced by olfactory stimuli with sexual connotations have been detected in homosexual men and women (Chapter 8).

These observations, performed initially in rats, were confirmed in mice, although in this species androgens themselves seem to play a more important role in the differentiation of sexual preferences. Christian Bodo, working in the laboratory of Emilie Rissman (University of Virginia), has shown that sexual differentiation is deeply disturbed in mice suffering from a mutation of the androgen receptor that prevents the action of testosterone or DHT (Bodo & Rissman, 2007). This mutation, called TFM for "testicular feminizing," has its equivalent in humans, as we shall see in Chapter 6. In behavioral tests performed on adult gonadectomized animals treated with estrogen to activate the behavior and sexual motivation, TFM male mice had responses similar to those of females for all characteristics that are sexually dimorphic and in which females typically differ from males. For example, in simultaneous choice tests, males spend more time investigating bedding soiled by the urine of females, while females and TFM males preferred bedding soiled by the urine of males. More females and TFM males showed no preference for one sex partner or another in choice tests while the control males showed a strong preference for a female partner. Finally, exposure to bedding soiled by males, but not to clean bedding, induced neuronal activation (measured by an induction of c-fos gene expression) in the preoptic area and the nucleus of the stria terminalis in females and TFM males but not in control males. Recent results from the same researchers also demonstrated that treatment of neonatal females with an androgen (dihydrotestosterone) masculinizes for life all these behavioral features and the response of the nervous system to male odors (Bodo & Rissman, 2008).

Studies with genetically engineered (knock-out, KO) mice that either lack the enzyme aromatase [and thus cannot synthesize estrogens, ArKO (Honda et al., 1998; Bakker et al., 2002b)] or do not express the alpha-fetoprotein [and are thus not protected from the masculinizing and defeminizing actions of maternal estrogens during embryonic life, AFPKO (Bakker et al., 2006)] similarly reveal a major impact of embryonic hormonal alterations on the sexual preferences of adult subjects. Because these altered preferences cannot usually be modified by adult endocrine treatments, it is assumed that they derive from organizational effects of steroids that took place in early life, even if this conclusion is often indirect and has not been formally demonstrated.

In a long series of experiments, Julie Bakker and collaborators analyzed the preferences displayed by male and female ArKO or AFPKO mice when presented with the opportunity to investigate body odors or cage bedding soiled by male or female stimuli. Studies with ArKO mice indicated that the development of sexual preferences in influenced by estrogens. Gonadally intact male ArKO mice (contrary to wild-type males) failed to show a preference for an estrous female versus a sexually active male when asked to discriminate between these stimuli based on volatile body odors (Bakker et al., 2002a). Accordingly, AFPKO females that are not protected from maternal estrogens during embryonic life display defeminized sexual behavior and partner preferences. They are unable to display lordosis behavior in adulthood (Bakker et al., 2006) and they show, contrary to wild-type females, a robust preference for an estrous female over an intact male when choosing between these stimuli based on volatile body odors (Bakker & Brock, 2010; Brock & Bakker, 2011). Together these data thus point to an important role of estrogens in the development of partner preference in mice. The relative role of estrogens (this section) vs. androgen (previous section) in the organization of these sexually differentiated characteristics remains to be established.

Together these findings thus support the idea that sexual preferences in mammals are controlled during ontogeny by the action of sex steroids, mainly estrogenic metabolites of testosterone in rats, possibly androgens and estrogens in mice. They are in agreement with clinical and correlative data suggesting the same conclusion in humans (see Chapters 8 and 9).

Finally, it is important to emphasize that these early hormonal manipulations seem to have absolutely irreversible effects on both the type of sexual behavior to be made in adulthood (male or female typical) and its orientation (homo- vs. heterosexual). So far, we have failed to find an experimental manipulation that would reverse in adulthood these behavioral characteristics induced by the hormonal milieu during embryonic or immediately postnatal life. In particular, the hormones secreted by adults are totally unable to change the type of sexual behavior expressed by an individual (male or female) and its orientation (homosexual or heterosexual). These animal studies play a critical role when we consider the potential hormonal basis of human homosexuality.

Most mammalian species, and in particular all those species that have been investigated in order to understand the endocrine controls of sexual preferences (rats, mice, ferrets, sheep), do not form stable pair bonds. This lack of stable bonds obviously prevents us from investigating this important aspect of sexual preference. In contrast, the majority of avian species form intersexual bonds that last either for one reproductive season or sometimes for the entire life. A highly relevant body of research has been carried out on the development of these sexual bonds in one songbird species, the zebra finch (*Taeniopygia guttata*) (summarized in Adkins-Regan, 2011). Zebra finches breed colonially but form socially monogamous heterosexual pairs at a young age that usually last until one member of the pair dies. Multiple behaviors that can be easily recorded attest the presence of this pair bond, such as clumping (perching in close contact), allopreening (preening each other), and spending time in a nest box together. These behaviors are observed almost exclusively within hetero-sexual pairs. Homosexual pairs do not occur in the wild and do so only rarely in captivity.

Although social context during rearing does affect partner preferences, these behaviors also seem to be controlled to a large extent by the action of steroids during development (organizational effect) but not in adulthood. Adult castra-tion or treatment with exogenous androgens or estrogens will eventually mod-ulate the expression of the behaviors indicative of pair bonding (decrease and activation of the behaviors, respectively) but will never modify their direction (toward a male or a female). The heterosexual direction of the sexual partner preference in zebra finches does not depend on the action of sex steroids in adulthood.

In contrast, if young females are treated with estrogens during the first two weeks posthatch, they will prefer other females over males in two-choice prox-imity tests and will pair with females in mixed-sex aviaries where they have ample choice of partners (Adkins-Regan & Ascenzi, 1987; Mansukhani et al., 1996; Adkins-Regan, 1999). It is quite interesting that this "homosexual" part-ner preference only develops if the estrogen-treated females are housed in all-female aviaries during their development. Neither all-female housing alone nor estrogen treatment alone produce a significant modification of the sexual part-ner preference. This finding obviously raises the question of what is actually modified by the treatment with estrogens. It has been speculated that the steroid masculinizes the way in which females learn (or become imprinted on) the sex of their partner, but additional work would be need to resolve this question.

These experiments therefore suggest that, in birds also, the action of steroids during development modify sexual preferences in a long-lasting manner. Interpretation of the results is complicated, however, by a number problems, including the facts (1) that the estrogen treatment that was used has been shown to display some toxicity and (2) that different treatments with aromatase inhibi-tor, which should decrease estrogen production and thus have an effect opposite to that of treatments increasing estrogen concentrations, also resulted in a shift from opposite-sex to same-sex preference in females and did not affect partner preferences in males (Adkins-Regan et al., 1996; Adkins-Regan & Wade, 2001). Similar paradoxical results have been previously reported during the experimental analysis of the sexual differentiation of singing activity and of the song control circuits in the zebra finch brain. Mechanisms mediating the sexual differentiation of brain and behavior in this species thus remain quite mysterious and clearly involve genetic effects that are not mediated by changes in gonadal steroid production (the so called "direct genetic effects," (Arnold et al., 2004; Arnold & Chen, 2009). More work will be needed on this topic but for the purpose of the present discussion, it should be noted that steroid action during ontogeny is able to affect the direction of partner preference in a long-lasting manner and the type of social bond that will be displayed by adult birds (see Adkins-Regan, 2011 for more details).

In conclusion, in animals that were studied, sexual orientation differentiates during ontogenesis under the influence of the same hormonal stimuli that differentiate the expression of motor behavior patterns. The embryonic or neonatal hormones determine not only the type of behavior that will be present in adulthood but also the subjects' homosexual or heterosexual orientation. Although social factors such as education and social environment must also potentially be taken into account, it seems that the biological (hormonal) factors described in animals also contribute to the determinism of sexual orientation in humans (see Chapters 8 and 9).

SEXUAL DIFFERENTIATION OF THE PREOPTIC AREA AND SEXUAL ORIENTATION IN THE RAT

It is also important to emphasize that the hormonal mechanisms that control the development of sexually differentiated brain structures such as the SDN of the preoptic area (see Chapter 3; Figure 3.7) are, in rats, similar to those that control the organization of orientation of sexual behavior and sexual performance. A newborn female rat treated early by testosterone possesses, in adulthood, a large volume of SDN similar to that of a control male and produces sexual behavior patterns typical of a male toward a female. Conversely, castration of a newborn male just after birth blocks the development of the SDN and inhibits masculinization of copulatory behavior (see Figure 3.7) (Jacobson et al., 1981; Arnold & Gorski, 1984). Finally, if male rats are injected during the end of their embryonic and early postnatal life with an aromatase inhibitor (which suppresses production of estrogen by aromatization of testosterone), in adulthood, these rats will be unable to show active copulatory behavior typical of the male and will present a partially reversed sexual orientation. They also possess at adult age a small SDN, characteristic of the female (Houtsmuller et al., 1994).

Recall that these effects of the hormonal environment on the organization of sexual behavior and its orientation, and on the size of the preoptic SDN, are observed only if the treatments occur during the critical period of sexual differentiation, which in rats covers the two weeks surrounding birth. The hormone treatments have important and irreversible effects if they are performed during that period, but no effect will be observed with later treatments.

That lesions of the preoptic area block the expression of male sexual behavior and reverse its orientation (see the beginning of this chapter) led to questions regarding the nature of links between the behavioral effects of early hormone treatments and their effects on the dimorphic nucleus of the preoptic area. Are the masculinization of behavior and changes in the size of the SDN caused by testosterone independent phenomena? Alternatively, does the effect of hormones on behavior lead to a change in the structure of the brain or, conversely, is the change in the brain at the basis of behavioral change?

It is well known that the expression of a behavior can induce changes in brain structure. For example, violinists have a particularly wide area in their motor cortex corresponding to the finger of the left hand that they use to block the strings on a violin (Elbert et al., 1995). Furthermore, rats reared in an enriched environment show a large number of physical changes in the brain (including an increased number of synapses, a more complex dendritic tree of neurons, and possibly a larger number of neurons). These environmental effects are probably more important for the development of the human brain than for the most primitive vertebrates, but it is very likely that the early hormonal effects on the size of the SDN induced by hormonal conditions in rats are directly responsible for the changes in the expression of behavior, rather than the reverse. It should be noted that the effects of perinatal treatment with testosterone can be observed in the young rat's brain development long before it reaches sexual maturity and begins to express copulatory behavior. It is therefore likely that changes in sexual behavior cannot be the basis of the effect on brain structure. This leaves only two possibilities: either the change of the brain governs the expression of behavior and orientation or both types of effects are induced in a more or less independent fashion by the early action of testosterone. Even in the most minimalist interpretation (the second one), the change in the volume of the SDN is at least a permanent physical signature of early androgen action that differentiated behavior. This signature has major documentary value, as the volume of the SDN is apparently not affected by the hormonal milieu of the adult animal. In rats, the volume of the SDN enables us to obtain retrospective information on the hormonal conditions under which an individual developed. We shall see later that this signature in the brain may play an important role in our interpretation of the mechanisms that potentially induce homosexuality in humans.

HOMOSEXUAL SHEEP

All the studies mentioned above describe animals that have certain aspects of what in humans is called a homosexual orientation. In all cases, however, note that it is almost never an exclusively homosexual orientation, only a homosexual preference in animals that are essentially bisexual. In addition, all animal models described so far relate to homosexual behavior induced experimentally, as opposed to behaviors that occur spontaneously. Over the past ten years, a spontaneous model of exclusive homosexuality has been described in sheep and is considered in detail here.

In studies of sexual behavior of male sheep, ethologists had early realized that the sexual capacity of rams is very variable. When presented with sexually receptive females, some males are capable of achieving as many as five or six ejaculations during a period of 30 minutes, while others are much less active or completely inactive in the presence of females (Resko et al., 1996; Pinckard et al., 2000). This sexual ability is obviously the object of special attention from farmers, as it makes some males much more productive breeding stock than others. Hundreds of males are studied each year in behavioral tests and, consistently, approximately 20% of rams do not qualify to be kept as breeding subjects in animal husbandry.

During more precise testing, it was noted that a significant fraction of these males with little or no reaction in the presence of females are in fact not completely asexual but have active sexual behavior if they are given another ram as sexual stimulus. During a quantitative study carried out on more than 700 rams, 51% of subjects offered a choice between a male or female partner oriented their behavior exclusively toward a female (male-oriented toward female; MOF), 31% were bisexual, 10% were asexual (did not present any behavior), and 8% oriented their sexual behavior exclusively toward another male (male-oriented male; MOM). The intensity of motivation and sexual performance among male-oriented males is not in question. It is specifically the focus of this behavior that is atypical.

Extensive studies were then carried out to identify the potential causes of this reversed sexual orientation (see Roselli et al., 2011 for review). It was first suggested that same-sex rearing, which is common in sheep, might promote the development of these MOM sheep. Comparisons between rams raised in mixed-sex groups and rams raised in all-male groups revealed small differences in young adults in the rate of mounting and ejaculations with estrous ewes, but most rams in both groups later developed a heterosexual mate preference. Also, a search by several independent groups for genetic determinations of sexual orientation did not provide any conclusive results and selection for reproduction in ewes did not affect sexual behavior or sexual orientation in male offspring.

Another idea put forward was that a differential sexual attraction might be related to the ability to process sensory, in particular olfactory, cues coming from the partner, and some limited support was obtained for this notion. Differential endocrine responses (increases in testosterone and/or luteinizing hormone concentrations) were detected following exposure to ewes in MOF and MOM (Perkins & Fitzgerald, 1992; Perkins et al., 1992) but some aspects of these studies make them difficult to interpret [see Roselli et al., (2011) for discussion]. Furthermore, brain activation, as measured by the induction of the protein product of the immediate early gene *fos*, was more intense in the medial preoptic area of MOF than of MOM, but this was observed after exposure to stimulus ewes as well as rams (Alexander et al., 1999). The difference observed might therefore relate to sexual orientation, as well as to an overall difference in brain activity. Together, available results indicate that none of these mechanisms are mutually exclusive, but none of them have been demonstrated conclusively to play a significant role. Attention then focused on potential differences in the preoptic area that could relate to sexual orientation.

Anatomical studies identified the existence of a sexually dimorphic nucleus in the preoptic area of sheep similar to that observed in rats. The sexually dimorphic nucleus of the sheep preoptic area (ovine SDN or oSDN) is approximately three times larger in males than in females (Figure 4.3) (Roselli et al., 2004b). The male oSDN has also about four times more neurons than that of females. It is interesting that the oSDN of the male-oriented male is significantly smaller than in the males oriented to females and contains significantly fewer neurons (Roselli et al., 2004a). It has a structure similar to that observed in females, with which male-oriented males share the same sexual orientation.

The sheep SDN is also characterized by a dense expression of aromatase. Quantitative studies of this enzyme in the preoptic area indicate that aromatase activity is higher in rams than in ewes, just as observed in rodents. In addition, aromatase activity in the preoptic area was significantly lower in male-oriented males than in males oriented to females, thus making them more similar to females (Roselli et al., 2004b). The volume of oSDN can also be measured by quantifying, in successive sections, the surface of dense expression of aromatase mRNA. This confirmed measurements of the oSDN obtained by conventional histological stains indicating that oSDN is larger in MOF than in females and MOM have an oSDN smaller than MOF.

These studies indicate that several characteristics of the preoptic area of rams (volume and number of neurons in the SDN, aromatase activity in the preoptic area) are correlated with sexual orientation (Perkins & Roselli, 2007). This correlation raises again the problem of the nature and direction of causal links between the volume and structure of oSDN and sexual behavior of rams. Does the oSDN control sexual orientation or does the orientation determine the size

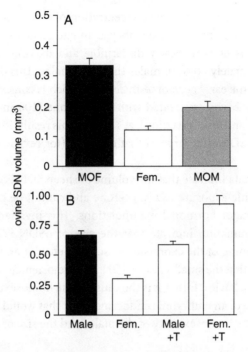

Figure 4.3 Volume of the sexually dimorphic nucleus of the preoptic area (oSDN) in sheep. A. oSDN volume is larger in males directed toward females (MOF) than among females (Fem.), but the male-oriented males (MOM) have a volume similar to that of females. B. Effect of treatment with testosterone between days 30 and 90 of gestation on the volume of oSDN measured at 135 days of gestation (birth at approximately 150 days). A significant increase in the volume of oSDN is observed among females but the same treatment has no effect in males [according to Roselli et al., (2004b) and Roselli et al. (2007)].

of the nucleus? The analysis of the hormonal mechanisms that control the development of the nucleus provides critical information on this topic.

If rams and ewes are gonadectomized in adulthood (castration of males and ovariectomy of females) and, after a month without hormone, all subjects are treated for three weeks with testosterone, at autopsy it can be shown that the size of the oSDN has not been changed by the manipulations. (The MOF oSDN remains about twice as large as in females and MOM SDN remains significantly smaller than that of MOF and thus similar to that of females.) These hormonal manipulations performed in adulthood suggest that the differentiation affecting the volume of oSDN precedes the establishment of sexual behavior and potentially its orientation. This idea has been confirmed by the analysis of the size of oSDN in embryos of sheep (Roselli et al., 2007). During the embryonic life of the sheep, which lasts about 150 days, between the 50th and 100th days of gestation there is a peak in the concentration of circulating testosterone in males that is not present in female embryos. In late gestation (days 135 to 140) the sheep SDN is already clearly discernible and its volume is significantly greater (approximately 60%) in males than in females. This difference is obviously caused by the early peak of testosterone, which is consistent with the fact that if female embryos are treated with testosterone (100 mg twice per week between days 30 and 90 of gestation), at 135 days this results in females in which the volume of oSDN is as large as that of males (for review see Roselli et al., 2011).

All available data indicate that the volume of sheep SDN is determined, as in rats, by embryonic exposure to testosterone and cannot be changed in adulthood even by major hormonal manipulations. This invariance in adulthood and early determination indicate that the size of oSDN is determined well before the beginning of the expression of sexual behavior and orientation. It is thus impossible that the small size of oSDN in male-oriented rams is the consequence of their behavior. Either it is the cause of the homosexual orientation or it is the signature of an embryonic endocrine event that would have determined independently the homosexuality of the males and the size of their oSDN.

IN CONCLUSION (IN PART . . .)

Recent research has identified neuroendocrine processes that control the differentiation and activation of many aspects of behavior in animals. Many questions remain open, particularly about how the hormones act at the cellular level in the brain. Although so far the bulk of research has been devoted to analyzing the mechanisms that control the sexual differentiation and activation of motor behavior patterns, interest has focused recently on the analysis, in animals, of other aspects of sexuality such as sexual orientation. This work has shown that this aspect of sexual behavior is largely controlled by the same hormones acting to a large extent on the same nervous sites as sexual performance.

It should be noted that, apart from the study of Henley and collaborators demonstrating an increase in preference for females in female rats injected with estradiol benzoate during the first three weeks of postnatal life (Henley et al., 2009), there have not been any studies devoted to the analysis of an animal model of female homosexuality. It is impossible to know whether this relative lack of data results from an experimental or technical difficulty or is simply the result of a sexist inclination on the part of researchers. It would be very interesting to test the sexual orientation of female sheep and rats androgenized during their prenatal or immediately postnatal life.

5

Gender Differences in Humans

MEN AND WOMEN ARE NOT IDENTICAL

In humans, as in most animal species, there are many physical, functional, and behavioral differences between the sexes. This means that in a quantitative study on a sufficient number of individuals, a statistically significant difference will be observed in the results obtained for men and women. This difference does not necessarily have a large amplitude or biological significance, but it is statistically significant—it is not simply the result of random fluctuations in the sample.

Physical sex differences, for example, concern not only the sexual organs (ovaries vs. testes; oviduct, uterus, vagina vs. seminiferous ducts, seminal vesicles, prostate; vulva and clitoris vs. scrotum and penis) but also various characters commonly classified under the term "secondary sexual characteristics" that include the presence of facial hair more developed in men (beard, mustache) or breasts in women. Neuroanatomical differences include a larger dimorphic nucleus of the preoptic area in males than in females, larger bed nucleus of the stria terminalis in males than in females, and greater thickness of the anterior commissure and of parts of the corpus callosum in females than in males.

Note also differences in circulating levels of various hormones (steroid sex hormones, obviously, but also hormones not directly related to reproduction), differences in various aspects of metabolism (pound for pound, men metabolize alcohol more quickly than women), and differences in susceptibility to various diseases, including diseases of the nervous system. Men are more frequently affected by autism (male:female incidence of 3:1) and schizophrenia (ratio of 2:1), while women are more often affected by depression (female:male = 2:1) and Alzheimer's disease (2:1) (Becker et al., 2008). Dyslexia is also twice as common among boys as girls in both Europe and the United States. At the behavioral level, differences between men and women are equally numerous. For example, men are on average significantly more aggressive than women. There are also reproducible cognitive differences between the sexes, but these are often of a lesser magnitude. For example, women have higher verbal skills (use of language and ability to spell words) than men, while men are better in certain aspects of mathematical reasoning and analysis of spatial relationships between objects.

The differences between men and women in physiology are, in fact, far too numerous to be summarized here. A very detailed book of 900 pages has been published recently on this issue, with references to more than 22,000 scientific studies on the subject (Ellis et al., 2008). The existence of such differences is not surprising when you consider that in animals (and probably in humans) most genes are differentially expressed between males and females. A recent study showed that in mice, 72% of genes expressed in the liver and 14% of genes expressed in the brain are different in males and females (Yang et al., 2006). The existence of differences between sexes may be the rule rather than the exception, even if the magnitude of these differences can vary greatly depending on the species and the character in question. Epidemiological or pharmacological studies would do well to take such differences into account more systematically, because many experimental results demonstrated in a population of one sex may well not apply directly to the other sex. A dose of medication that is effective and safe in one sex may be less effective or have side effects in the other sex [see the Web site of the Organization for the Study of Sex Differences (OSSD) at www://http.ossdweb.org].

BIOLOGY OR EDUCATION?

It is clear that the primary physical sex differences are due almost exclusively to early hormonal influences. As noted in the previous section, the fusion of genital folds into a scrotum and the development of the genital tubercle in a penis are induced in the animal embryo (rats, mice) by the action of testosterone, which must be transformed into dihydrotestosterone (DHT) by the action of 5α-reductase to exert these physical effects. The same is true in humans (see Chapter 6). Well-known disturbances of these processes, observed either in individuals with androgen insensitivity (due to a mutation in the receptor to testosterone and DHT) or in subjects deficient in 5α-reductase, demonstrate the critical influence of hormones in determining these sex differences, even in humans. Affected individuals are born with partially or completely female genitals depending on the magnitude of the clinical problem. It is most unlikely that any aspect of the environment could be influencing such hormonal actions.

Some physical characteristics are more labile (that is, they are variable, unlike the external genital structures that are determined in their more or less final form before birth), and although they are markedly controlled by the sex steroids, they are also affected by the environment. For example, breasts are normally a female secondary sexual characteristic, but accidental exposure to overly high quantities of estrogen (by, for example, consumption of poultry meat contaminated with these hormones) can induce their growth in boys.

Other differences may have physiological determinism that more or less equally includes biological and environmental factors. It is clear that in a Western population, the increased capacity that men have to metabolize alcohol compared to women may result partly from a differential expression of genes in the liver (74% of genes expressed by the liver are expressed differently in male and female mice) (Yang et al., 2006), but also from the fact that men generally drink more alcohol than women and more frequent consumption of alcohol stimulates greater production of the enzymes that metabolize alcohol.

Finally, in many other cases, gender differences are mainly a reflection of past experiences of the individual. Education, activities, and the expectations of society and parents indeed vary depending on the sex of a child. Given the importance of learning phenomena in humans, it is not surprising that all these factors have a profound effect on the development of differences between sexes. This is particularly the case for many differences in behavior and cognitive skills, but that does not mean that there is not in parallel some biological contribution to these differences.

THE DIFFERENCES OF SEXUAL BEHAVIOR: VARIABLE AMPLITUDE AND THE DIFFICULTY OF IDENTIFYING ORIGIN

The interaction between biological and environmental determinism is particularly complex when it comes to control mechanisms of behavior in humans. Many differing aspects of behavior are noted along gender lines. For example, it is widely accepted (at least in Western societies) that women have more developed skills in verbal communication whereas men perform better in tasks involving mathematical reasoning or mental visualization of the rotation of an object. These differences have been systematically studied in controlled populations and confirmed statistically (e.g., Benbow, 1993).

However, these differences are very much rooted in the different educations received by boys and girls. This idea is particularly supported by recent data

indicating that gender differences in math skills have greatly reduced or can-
celed, or even reversed, during the last 20 to 30 years, which have also seen an
increase in girls' access to higher education in Western countries (Guiso et al.,
2008; Hyde et al., 2008). The intercultural comparison also shows that the more
societies treat boys and girls equally, particularly in education, the more the
difference in math ability is reduced (Guiso et al., 2008). Quite unexpectedly,
however, this more equal treatment for boys and girls increases the difference
in reading ability that already favored girls. It seems that girls have an inher-
ently higher ability to read than boys do, but that difference is partly hidden in
societies where girls are less educated than boys and is fully revealed when we
offer girls an equal opportunity to develop their capacities (Guiso et al., 2008).

It must be pointed out that the magnitude of these differences is generally
very low and there is an overlap between the performances of individuals of
both sexes. Statisticians have developed a tool to quantify and compare differences between populations. This measure is the effect size. Consider the distribution of scores (see Figure 5.1) obtained by a group of men (light gray) and
women (dark gray) on a psychological test measuring a sexually differentiated
behavior or any physical variable in both sexes. The magnitude of sex differences involved is very different in the two cases that are illustrated. The size of
the effect is simply the ratio of the difference between mean values observed in
both groups (DM, DM') to the common standard deviation of samples (SD,
SD'), a measure of the average variance within these groups.

The difference between averages (DM) is relatively important in the case
illustrated on the left, while this difference is small on the right (DM'). The variability between subjects within the same group remains more or less the same
(SD = ± SD'). The size of an effect is especially important when the ratio of DM
to SD or DM' to SD' is large. The size of the effect is considered large if greater
than 0.8, moderate for values between 0.8 and 0.2, and small or negligible for
lower values (< 0.2). When the size of an effect is large (left figure), the score of

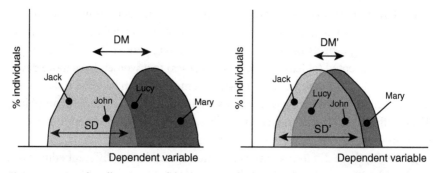

Figure 5.1 Graphic illustration of the concept of effect size (according to Nelson, 2005).

an individual can predict his or her sex with a good probability (Lucy and Mary have scores higher than Jack and John), but this is no longer the case for small effect sizes. On the right side of the figure, John has a higher score than Lucy for the variable concerned, while men have an average score lower than women.

The effect size of "sex differences" for many physical variables is large (> 0.8). This is true for measures such as the height of an individual but also for neuro-anatomical differences such as that affecting the volume of the dimorphic nucleus of the preoptic area. This nucleus is indeed about two times larger in men than in women (Swaab & Fliers, 1985). In contrast, the differences in cognitive abilities (e.g., verbal overall capacity) are often more limited and effect sizes very often described as low to negligible (< 0.2). There are exceptions. For example, mental rotation skill of three-dimensional objects is associated with a sex difference that is considered large (> 0.8, see Figure 5.2).

Many differences in cognitive skills (e.g., mathematical reasoning, verbal ability, spatial perception) have a low amplitude, even if they are reproducible. They can be identified by statistics in a relatively large population, but the overlap of distribution curves is large, so it is not possible to determine the sex of an individual from his score on one of these tests. In everyday life, there is no reason to tolerate any discrimination between the sexes for such tasks. Even if a job requires a skill known to be sexually differentiated, and for which men are

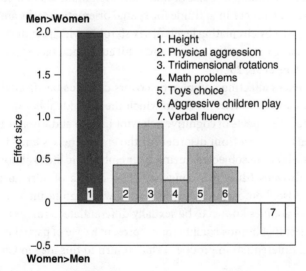

Figure 5.2 Magnitude of sex differences affecting various human characteristics. The amplitude is measured by the effect size (difference between means divided by the variance of the population). Positive values indicate differences in favor of men, negative values represent differences in favor of women. The effect size is large (> 0.8) for physical differences but generally low for behavioral or cognitive differences, except for the difference in the ability to rotate three-dimensional objects (according to Hines, 2004).

on average more efficient, it is very likely to be found in women candidates for the position who are better than male candidates (and vice versa). Any discrimination based on sex is not justified by the existence of statistical differences of the small magnitude that we are talking about here.

Some authors have sought to demonstrate, either for ideological reasons or to counter existing discrimination, that the behavioral differences that I have mentioned do not exist (e.g., Vidal, 2000; Vidal, 2007). I believe that this is a false battle. The fight against discrimination is laudable, but it will be more effective if it is based on a correct analysis of the real situation. There are obvious behavioral differences between men and women. The real question is this: Is their origin biological (genetic, hormonal) or environmental (education, social)? It is obvious that these differences are induced to a large extent by differently focused educations given to boys and girls. However, this does not necessarily mean that certain biological influences are not also involved in their determinism.

The equivalent of a verbal or mathematical reasoning can hardly be studied in animals, but there are very similar cognitive behaviors present in animals and humans for which the control mechanisms can be more easily analyzed. For example, it is generally observed in spatial orientation tasks that male rodents have superior performance to those of females. This difference recalls sex differences affecting orientation in space that have been identified in humans in some studies, although the size of this effect in humans is small. It was shown that these sex differences in aptitude for spatial orientation tasks are controlled in rodents in part by circulating levels of sex steroids, which act during development (organizing irreversible effects) and until adulthood (activation transitory effects) (Imwalle et al., 2006).

Sex differences affecting complex behaviors can thus be affected in parallel by hormones and the environment in which the individual has developed. We will see that some aspects of cognitive behavior in men and women are changed in individuals suffering from disorders of the endocrine system—for example, among girls who were subjected during their embryonic life to abnormally high levels of androgens (due to a congenital hyperplasia of adrenal glands, see Chapter 6). Also, homosexuality is associated with significant changes in certain cognitive abilities known to be sexually differentiated. This association was used to suggest that homosexuality may represent a case of partial modification of the sexual differentiation process. I shall return to this idea in Chapter 8.

SEXUAL ORIENTATION AND IDENTITY ARE THE MOST DIFFERENTIATED BEHAVIORAL CHARACTERISTICS

In this chapter, I have briefly reviewed the different physical, functional, and behavioral characteristics that have been shown to be sexually differentiated in humans. The magnitude of these differences is highly variable. At the behavioral level in particular, the size of differences in statistical terms is small. As one might expect, it is in the sexual area that the largest differences between genders are observed. Sexual orientation and sexual identity (two different aspects of human sexuality that should not be confounded; see Chapter 1 for detailed discussion) are without a doubt the most sexually differentiated characteristics in humans. In the majority of the population (over 90%) there is indeed usually no overlap between the sexual orientation of men and women. Homosexuality in this context represents the absence of difference between sexes for "sexual orientation." A gay man displays sexual attraction for individuals of the same sex as a heterosexual woman does. Conversely, homosexual women show sexual preferences for women just as heterosexual males do. The specific individual(s) that will be selected as partner(s) might admittedly be different in these categories (men found attractive by a gay men might not be attractive to a women), but it remains that in homosexual subjects there is a reversal of the sex that is considered sexually attractive.

This sex difference has a remarkable consistency throughout the world and among different cultures, independently of whether they are very or somewhat tolerant vis-à-vis homosexuality (see Chapter 1). It is only in societies where homosexuality is severely punished that the official statistics indicate a complete absence of homosexuals. However, once the political regime changes in these countries, in less than a generation the gay population corresponds to what is observed in the rest of the world.

The difference between sexes is even more marked at the level of sexual identity. The number of transsexuals, that is, individuals of one sex who think themselves to be of the opposite sex, is even lower (well below 1%). U.S. estimates are that 1 in 30,000 men and 1 in 1,00,000 women seek medical treatment and surgery to change sex. Less important disorders of sexual identity, including the desire to be of the opposite sex but falling short of demanding surgery, are probably more frequent, but accurate statistics are difficult to obtain. Statistics from the Netherlands, where medical and psychological help is widely available for patients suffering from sexual identity problems, indicate the presence of these disorders in about 1 man out of 20,000 and 1 woman in 50,000 (Hines, 2004). These disorders remain rare exceptions, and the vast majority of men and women self-identify as such.

We are entitled to ask what the mechanisms are that lead to the establishment of a difference so stable and reproducible between men and women, even if there are "rare" exceptions. It is clear from an evolutionary point of view that these characteristics are extremely important, as they are closely related to reproductive success and the sustainability of the species and therefore more directly to the transmission to the next generation of combinations of genes that support them (if they exist). Sexual orientation itself is highly differentiated between males and females in most species that reproduce sexually (gender identity does not exist or is impossible to study in animals). One could imagine that the human species has invented a new way, based on learning, to ensure that men and women have an orientation and therefore a sexual attraction toward the opposite sex, thus ensuring successful reproduction. However, it is worth considering in such circumstances the famous logical rule of thumb called Occam's razor (also known as "law of parsimony"): "Entities must not be multiplied beyond necessity"—in other words, the simplest explanation is likely to be the best one. The simplest explanation is that the mechanisms existing in animals have been transmitted to humans, even if cultural controls, unidentified so far, have been added.

6

The Effects of Sex Steroids in Humans

Organizing Effects

THE NATURE OF THE EXPERIMENTAL EVIDENCE: CORRELATION IS NOT CAUSATION

In Chapters 3 and 4 I reviewed many of the principles highlighted in various animal models on the effects of sex steroids on the expression of reproductive behavior, on sexual differentiation during development, and on the sexual orientation. I now examine the available data suggesting that these mechanisms are still active in the human species.

The nature of the data that suggest that similar mechanisms are found in animals and in humans is quite different. In animals, conclusions are based primarily on experimental studies. In general, a population of experimental subjects is randomly divided into two or more subgroups that are then subjected to two or more experimental treatments. For example, 20 rats are castrated and 10 of them receive a daily injection of testosterone while the other 10 are injected with oil in which testosterone is dissolved. After one or two weeks, during standardized tests in which males are in the presence of a sexually receptive female, the subjects treated with testosterone show active sexual behavior whereas the control subjects injected with oil are inactive. This experiment demonstrates that injecting testosterone causes the activation of sexual behavior in male rats.

We have excellent reasons to believe that the same is true in humans; however, the nature of the data supporting this conclusion is different. For obvious ethical reasons, performing a castration in humans purely for experimental purposes is forbidden, or even to treat subjects chronically with testosterone. Beyond that, there are obvious methodological difficulties associated with obtaining a reliable measure of human sexual behavior. The data indicate, however, that male sexual behavior of the human species is, as in rats, influenced by testosterone. The arguments supporting this argument are threefold.

Comparison with animal species provides a first type of argument. It is known that human testes produce testosterone identical to that secreted in rodents such as rats and mice and in most vertebrates. Testosterone circulates in the blood of adult humans at concentrations similar to those observed in other vertebrates, and postmortem anatomical studies have shown that the human brain has receptors for testosterone similar to those of rats or monkeys, and these receptors are located in exactly the same areas of the brain (Abdelgadir et al., 1999; Fernández-Guasti et al., 2000; Pelletier, 2000; Kruijver et al., 2001). This argument is somewhat indirect and may only convince biologists, but it is strongly reinforced by the analysis of various clinical cases and the outcome of their medical treatment.

These clinical studies provide a second type of argument, much more direct, although they are prone to problems of interpretation. For example, there are human cases of clearly insufficient development of the testes that produce very low levels of circulating testosterone (less than 10% of values considered normal). Some of these patients consult endocrinology clinics because they complain of various sexual disorders, including a lack of desire and sexual motivation, a lack of erotic fantasies, and weak erections. Clinical studies conducted in controlled conditions have shown that treatment of these patients with testosterone significantly increased all measures of activity and sexual motivation, such as the number of nocturnal erections, thoughts and sexual fantasies, and masturbation episodes (Davidson et al., 1979; Bancroft, 1995; Hajjar et al., 1997; Snyder et al., 2000; Wang et al., 2000). Conversely, pharmacological manipulations that lower levels of circulating testosterone induce a decrease in libido and various aspects of sexual behavior in humans (Rosler & Witztum, 1998). These studies are generally carried out in double-blind conditions in which patients are treated either by testosterone or by a control solution (vehicle injection), and neither the doctor nor the patient knows during the study period who received testosterone or placebo. These studies demonstrate as clearly as possible in humans the behavioral effects of sex steroids. It must be pointed out that the conclusions that can be drawn from such studies are not necessarily generalizable to other physiological situations. For example, other forms of sexual disability will not be improved by added testosterone if there is not initially a very low circulating level.

In addition, there are many questions that can only be definitively answered with experiments that are unethical to carry out on humans, in particular the detection of brain sites where steroids act to activate the behavior. For such questions, studies are limited in humans to the use of a third strategy, namely, analysis of correlations between accidental brain damage and behavioral and endocrine/physiological variables. When a correlation has been established, its meaning must be sought by other methods, including comparison with animal studies.

A correlation between two variables does not in fact demonstrate that they are linked by a direct causal relationship. For example, if we observe that a particular behavioral characteristic such as frequency of sexual fantasies is correlated with the level of circulating testosterone (either within different individuals at one time or in an individual over time), it is possible either that testosterone stimulates behavior, or behavior activates the secretion of testosterone, or that the two variables are stimulated or inhibited by a third independent variable, such as the level of stress or relaxation of the individual. Only further studies can help interpret the observed correlation.

A substantial part of this book is devoted to a review of various types of physical, functional, and behavioral variables that correlate with homosexuality. These correlations can be interpreted schematically in three ways: either variable A is the cause of homosexuality (case 1), or the appearance of A is the result of homosexuality (case 2), or A and homosexuality are both the result of a cause that remains to be identified (case 3). It should be noted that these interpretations are not mutually exclusive and a variable can, for example, represent a partial cause of homosexuality but at the same time be reinforced by the expression of this sexual orientation (simultaneous occurrence of cases 1 and 2). In the absence of experimental studies that manipulate the incidence of homosexuality in a given population (ethically prohibited, obviously), the interpretation of these correlations will remain somewhat uncertain. The presence of these correlations, however, clarifies and restricts the possible causes of homosexuality. This is particularly the case if multiple correlations are considered in parallel and if one compares these results with those of animal studies. It is clear that only cases 1 and 3 are likely to explain the origins of homosexuality. Condition 2 reveals only a more or less direct consequence of this orientation. Throughout the following discussion I shall try to clarify the potential causal significance of various characteristics to be analyzed. In many cases, this meaning is not known with certainty, so I shall discuss the relative likelihood of each of these solutions.

The remainder of this section is devoted to a brief review of the available evidence that is consistent with the concept and demonstrates in many cases that the effects of steroid hormones that have been identified in animals are also present in humans, although they are sometimes partially masked by other mechanisms. The human species is indeed the result of a long evolution, and there is no reason to believe that the mechanisms of endocrine control of behavior that have been identified in fish and mammals—and are still quite evident in primates— have completely disappeared in our species. I obviously do not deny the specificity of the human species. But as much as it is characterized by a spectacular development of the cerebral cortex that has taken control over virtually all aspects of behavior, this does not exclude the survival of more primitive underlying biological mechanisms. I consider first the biological mechanisms of sex determination that are identical in animals and in humans. I then consider the current state of knowledge on the organizing and activating effects of sex steroids on physical and behavioral characteristics.

THE SEX DETERMINATION IN HUMANS

At an early stage of development, the embryonic gonad or germinal ridge is undifferentiated and bipotential. The subsequent development of the gonad into testis or ovary is determined by the cellular expression or absence of a protein, called testis-determining factor or TDF, encoded by the SRY gene present on chromosome Y (Berta et al., 1990; Sinclair et al., 1990). Sex determination in humans, as in mammals, takes place following entrance into the egg of a sperm with a X or Y chromosome.

The TDF protein then regulates the expression of many genes, leading to central cell proliferation at the expense of outermost layers of the germinal ridge so that the previously undifferentiated gonad develops into a testis. If an individual does not possess the Y chromosome (or has it, but the SRY gene is defective), the TDF protein is not produced and development of the embryonic gonad does not lead to the formation of a testis. In the presence of additional signals, ovaries will be formed. Once differentiated, the gonads influence sexual differentiation through their hormone production.

The data relating to the human species clearly indicate that the same mechanisms are involved as in animals during differentiation of the germinal ridge into a testis or ovary. Besides XY men and XX women, there are indeed people who have additional sex chromosome. XXY, XXYY, XYY, or XXX and X0 (the 0 indicates the absence of a second sexual chromosome) individuals have been identified in humans. The first group of anomalies of sex chromosomes (XXY, XXYY, XYY) is invariably associated with a male phenotype, whereas the second group (X0 and XXX) always produces female individuals. In other words, almost any embryo that has at least one Y chromosome develops as male and almost anyone who does not have a Y develops as female regardless of the other chromosomes that are present (but see below). This observation, coupled with what we knew of sexual differentiation in animals, led doctors to postulate as early as the 1950s that the Y chromosome includes a gene that determines the sex of the embryo.

The identification of this gene had to await progress in molecular biology and was carried out forty years later.

The British group of Andrew Sinclair was able to take advantage of the detailed study of a small group of individuals in which the correlation between the presence/absence of a Y chromosome and the man/woman phenotype is not present (Sinclair et al., 1990). There are indeed very rare cases in which there is a male phenotype in XX individuals and, vice versa, a female phenotype in XY individuals. Researchers have found that in XX men, a small fragment of the Y chromosome was transposed (translocated in scientific terms) on the X chromosome. This translocation occurs exceptionally in one of the cell divisions that lead to the formation of sperm. A small piece of chromosome "breaks" and joins erroneously to another chromosome, here the X chromosome. Conversely, there are a few individuals with XY chromosomes that have a female phenotype. In these individuals, the same small piece of the Y chromosome was broken and was lost during the production of sperm. By studying the DNA contained in this little piece of Y chromosome that when lost or translocated produces a reverse sex, British researchers were able to identify in humans the SRY (sex-determining region of the Y chromosome) gene that encodes the information to produce the protein TDF (testis-determining factor), which then determines the sex of the individual. The few cases of translocation or loss of this gene clearly confirm its key role in humans and animals.

The equivalent gene (SRY) exists in mice, and experimental evidence of the role of SRY in humans is linked in part to the comparison with the animal (see Chapter 3). By genetic manipulations, it has been demonstrated in mice that specific deletion of the SRY gene leads to the development of subjects that have a completely female phenotype even though the rest of their genetic sex is male. Conversely the "graft" on a non–sex chromosome of a female of the SRY gene produces a female that will develop testes, and the hormones secreted by the testes will masculinize the physical, functional, and behavioral traits of the subject (De Vries et al., 2002; Arnold & Chen, 2009).

ORGANIZING EFFECTS OF STEROIDS ON PHYSICAL AND BEHAVIORAL TRAITS IN HUMANS

Physical Traits

In the embryonic stage, all individuals have the tissues that are the precursors of male and female reproductive tracts. Thus the fetus at an early stage has a genital tubercle that can form either a penis or a clitoris and the genital folds that can form the lips of the vulva in females or testicular scrotum in males (Figure 3.5). At an early stage, the embryo also contains two sets of ducts that connect the gonads to the outside of the body: the Wolffian and Müllerian ducts (Figure 3.4).

In humans as in other male mammals, testosterone produced by Leydig cells of fetal testes causes the differentiation of Wolffian ducts into epididymis, vas deferens, and seminal vesicles. Sertoli cells will produce a peptide hormone, the anti-Müllerian hormone, or AMH, which as its name suggests, induces rapid and complete regression of Müllerian ducts (Figure 3.4).

In the female embryo, the ovary secretes little or no steroid hormones. The production of testosterone is virtually absent, and if estradiol is produced, it is in low concentrations that will bind to a circulating embryonic protein called alpha-fetoprotein that prevents the action of the steroid at the intracellular level. Consequently, Müllerian ducts spontaneously develop while Wolffian ducts regress completely. Sexual differentiation of the internal reproductive organs takes place along two independent axes: (1) demasculinization-masculinization and (2) defeminization-feminization. For normal development of the male reproductive system, the embryonic organ precursors undergo defeminizing hormonal effects (regression of Müllerian ducts by anti-Müllerian hormone produced in Sertoli cells) and masculinizing effects (development of Wolffian ducts promoted by testosterone). The female reproductive tract will appear as a result of feminization (development of Müllerian ducts) and demasculinization (regression of Wolffian ducts) and does not depend a priori on any hormone production. This dual mechanism directs the main changes leading to the acquisition of physical gender.

While the internal reproductive organs differentiate through development and regression of two separate drafts originally present in both sexes, this is not the case for the external genitalia. They differentiate in effect from the same embryonic structures (the genital tubercle and genital folds). Depending on whether testosterone is or is not present at a critical stage, these will change in the male or female external genitalia (Figure 3.5). The presence of testosterone [specifically its androgenic metabolite, 5α-dihydrotestosterone (DHT) produced by the enzyme 5α-reductase], induces the development of the male external genitals by fusion of the folds to form a scrotum and the development of the genital tubercle to form a penis. In the absence of testosterone, the genital folds do not fuse and instead form the vaginal lips, while the genital tubercle develops only slightly and turns into a clitoris. The same result is obtained in the absence of gonad. Thus, in humans, as in other mammals, hormone production is not required for normal development of the female reproductive system; hence it is generally regarded as the "default" developing sex or neutral sex.

This difference between the development of internal and external structures has important implications for individuals exposed for various reasons to abnormal hormonal conditions. In a series of clinical conditions, it is indeed theoretically possible to obtain adults who possess in parallel the internal sexual organs typical of the male and female. In contrast, external structures are more or less male or female but never both. The genital tubercle can develop to varying degrees ranging from a "normal" clitoris to a "normal" penis through all stages of more or less enlarged clitoris, but there is never the simultaneous presence of two types of structures, since they derive from the same embryonic tissue.

Behavioral Traits

It should also be noted that the principles that apply to sexual differentiation of the anatomy of the reproductive system in animals and in humans are also involved in the emergence of many differences affecting sexual behavior. It is clearly established in animals that typical male behaviors are generated by masculinization of the male under the influence of embryonic testosterone. Typical female behavior is present in the absence of hormones, but typical female behavior would be lost following embryonic exposure to testosterone (defeminization). Typical male and female behaviors can be considered as independent entities that depend heavily on different areas of the brain. It is therefore conceivable that these two types of behavior can persist simultaneously in an adult individual, and this condition has been observed in animals subjected to specific hormonal treatment during their development. Sexual differentiation of behavior does not occur, therefore, along a single axis from more masculine to more feminine, but along two more or less independent axes involving structures controlling male and female behavior. We shall see later how these concepts can be applied to the human species.

PHYSICAL CONSEQUENCES OF ENDOCRINE ABNORMALITIES IN HUMAN EMBRYOS

Experiments conducted in animals (mainly rats and mice but also monkeys) have clearly established the role played by testosterone in sexual differentiation of internal and external sex organs. Numerous clinical studies confirm that the mechanisms described in the previous section are also valid in humans, in whom testosterone plays a critical role in the development of sex organs of male embryos. Several diseases in the embryo that affect either the concentrations of circulating testosterone or the action of this steroid at the cellular level have been characterized in detail. They are invariably associated with atypical development of external genitalia and internal structures. I describe some of these diseases here, because they demonstrate the profound role steroids play in human development. Furthermore, these pathologies are also associated with behavioral changes that I discuss in Chapter 9. Four types of diseases or clinical conditions will be useful to examine in this context. The first two specifically affect boys, the next two concern girls.

The Androgen Insensitivity of XY Embryos

To exert its physical and behavioral effects, testosterone binds to specific intracellular receptors, the androgen receptors. These receptors are proteins that, when occupied by testosterone, partially change structure and interact with DNA to stimulate or suppress the synthesis of various mRNAs, which are then translated into proteins that influence the cellular function. Hundreds of mutations of the androgen receptor (changes in the structure of the corresponding gene) have been described. These mutations lead to production of a receptor protein that is either completely unable to fix testosterone or else fixes it with a lower affinity. The result is a complete or partial insensitivity to androgens (androgen insensitivity syndrome, AIS) whereby testosterone and other androgens are unable to induce their physical, functional, and behavioral effects. It is estimated that one child in 10,000 is affected by AIS, which is also incorrectly called testicular feminization syndrome. The androgen receptor gene is located on chromosome X.

If a woman who carries the AIS syndrome in heterozygotic state (presence of the mutation on one of the two X chromosomes) has an XY baby, there is one chance in two that he will be affected by the syndrome. In this genetic male, testes develop under the influence of the SRY gene and often produce normal secretion of testosterone and of the anti-Müllerian hormone that induces regression of Müllerian ducts (no development of oviduct or of uterus). Testosterone has no effect, however. Depending on the specific mutation (complete vs. partial AIS), internal genital structures derived from Wolfian ducts (e.g., epididymis) will or will not be present. More conspicuously, the genital tubercle and genital folds continue their development in the absence of testosterone action, as in a typical anhormonal state normally present in female embryos. The tubercle remains small and forms a clitoris, and the genital folds do not merge and instead form the lips of the vulva (no testicular scrotum). External genitalia of these individuals will be typically female at birth (Figure 6.1).

AIS XY girls are sometimes diagnosed at birth because of the presence of a blind vagina or because the testes are palpable under the skin in the genital area, where they remained blocked because testicular descent cannot complete in the absence of a scrotum. Many cases are not identified and are simply accepted as normal girls.

In summary, although male-typical hormones are present in normal concentrations in AIS XY subjects, testosterone is completely unable to act and

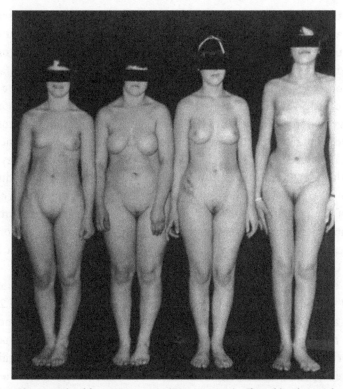

Figure 6.1 Photograph of four XY women (XY genotype) affected by the syndrome of androgen insensitivity (AIS). Presumably normal levels of testosterone were present in these individuals during embryonic life but could not act due to the mutation of the androgen receptor. Completely female morphology has therefore developed. (Google Image Search, AIS syndrome).

masculinize embryos. Their phenotype (appearance) will be entirely female. This extremely precise disorder affects only one specific protein, the androgen receptor, which very clearly demonstrates the effects of testosterone during development and effectively illustrates the crucial role of this steroid on the development of sexual morphology. Also note that the lack of masculinization of male embryos affected by the androgen insensitivity is accompanied by significant behavioral changes that affect both gender identity and sexual orientation. I return to this in later chapters.

5α-Reductase Deficiency in the Young Boy

As explained in the section on sexual differentiation in animals, testosterone must be converted into 5α-dihydrotestosterone (DHT) in the skin of the genital area to promote growth of the male external sexual structures (development of the genital tubercle into a penis and fusion of genital folds to form a scrotum). DHT is an androgen more potent than testosterone and is the only one capable of masculinizing external genital structures; the embryonic testosterone concentration is insufficient to achieve this result.

The conversion of testosterone into DHT is catalyzed (promoted) by a protein enzyme called 5α-reductase, which is expressed at high levels in the genital tubercle and genital folds. In the early 1970s, Imperato-McGinley and her colleagues identified a mutation of the 5α-reductase enzyme that makes it functionally unable to produce DHT (Imperato-McGinley, 1994; Imperato-McGinley & Zhu, 2002). This mutation in the gene controlling the production of 5α-reductase is recessive. It is only visible when present in a homozygous state (on both chromosomes of the pair). It has been observed in island societies where circumstances make inbreeding unusually common; it was first discovered in the Dominican Republic, but cases have been found subsequently in Papua New Guinea, Europe, and the United States.

Male embryos (XY chromosomes) affected by this mutation are born with external genital structures only partially masculinized (see Figure 6.2). They develop apparently normal testes that secrete the anti-Müllerian hormone that induces regression of structures derived from Müllerian ducts (fallopian tubes and uterus). Testosterone also promotes the development of internal sexual structures typical of the male, but at the level of external genitalia, the genital

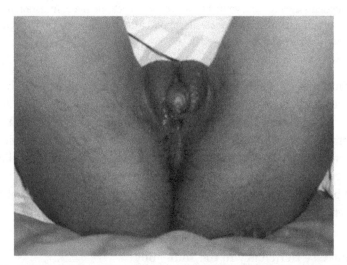

Figure 6.2 Genital structures not masculinized in an XY individual (male) suffering from a deficiency in 5α-reductase. Figure taken from Mishra, Reddy, and Chaturvedi (Bombay Hospial Journal 46/02, Case #23), reproduced with permission of P. Kapoor, Editor of the *Bombay Hospital Journal*.

tubercle either doesn't develop or develops very little and remains about the size of a clitoris. There is no fusion of genital folds: we observe at birth the presence of lips surrounding an opening to a blind vagina. There is therefore no scrotum, and testes are located under the skin around the lips of the blind genital opening or in the inguinal canal.

In adolescence, dramatic increases in the circulating levels of testosterone induce a partial masculinization of the genital structures. The skin of the genital folds' wrinkles darkens so it looks more like a scrotum, the testicles will continue their descent and will be found in the genital folds, and the genital tubercle will develop somewhat to resemble a small penis. The opening of the urethra remains on the base of the "penis," a medical condition called hypospadias. Pubertal male testosterone also affects various other physical aspects: It will increase the muscles and lower the tone of the voice. From a superficial point of view, these individuals look as though they have changed sex at least partially.

Male individuals affected by this change are essentially raised as girls and adopt a female sexual identity during childhood. In communities that are familiar with this syndrome, affected boys are clearly identified at birth, however, and the local language has a specific term to designate them (*Guevedoche* in the Dominican Republic, which in Spanish means "eggs," i.e., testes, and "twelve years"; or *Kwolu-aatmwol* in Papua, which means "female thing transforming into male thing"). One can imagine that those affected are to some extent considered intersex individuals. Intersex morphology at birth and partial change of sex morphology at puberty are also associated with the changes in identity and sexual role that I shall discuss in following sections.

Congenital Adrenal Hyperplasia in the Female Embryo

Congenital hyperplasia (excessive development) of the adrenal glands (CAH) is a genetic disorder that affects one of the enzymes involved in the synthesis of corticosteroid hormones (cortisol) from cholesterol (often 17α- or 21-hydroxylase). This synthesis of cortisol occurs in the adrenal glands. Cortisol is an important hormone involved in immune responses, carbohydrate metabolism, and response to stress. It is therefore not directly related to reproduction, but if its production is interrupted by genetic defect (e.g., CAH), one observes in response a hypersecretion of androgens (compounds similar to testosterone) in the affected embryos (Hines, 2003; MacLaughlin & Donahoe, 2004).

CAH syndrome is an autosomal recessive disease (carried by non–sex chromosomes). If both parents carry one defective copy of the gene, each of their children, regardless of sex, will have one chance out of four to have two copies of the mutated gene and be affected. It is estimated that one child in 16,000 is affected by this syndrome. If the affected fetus is male, additional androgens secreted by the adrenal gland will have little influence because they are simply added to the large amounts of androgens produced by the testicles. In addition to the metabolic problems associated with the absence of cortisol, we observe in affected female individuals a more or less profound masculinization of the external genital structures. In the most severely affected individuals, the genital tubercle has developed into a fully formed penis with a size almost equal to that seen in male babies. In addition there is a more or less complete fusion of the genital lips that form a scrotum (Figure 6.3). There are, of course, no testicles. The sex of these children is female. SRY is absent and consequently ovaries are formed. The anti-Müllerian hormone was not produced and the Wolffian ducts have developed into a uterus and oviducts. The internal reproductive organs are those of normal girls.

This more or less complete masculinization of external genital structures in CAH girls is usually detected at birth. These children will be treated during their entire life by administration of glucocorticoids. This treatment, by feedback on the activity of the pituitary, also suppresses the pathological production of androgens by the adrenal glands. Masculinized external genital structures are often "corrected" surgically, removing part of the penis to reproduce the clitoris and incising the genital folds to reopen the vaginal opening. These children are then raised as girls as far as we can know. From a scientific point of

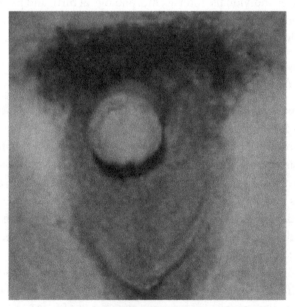

Figure 6.3 Genital structures in a masculinized XX individual (female) suffering from adrenal hyperplasia (CAH). Image from Legros J.J. et al. 1974. *Revue Médicale de Liège* 29, February 1974, pp. 73–80; reproduced with permission.

view, CAH girls allow one to assess, as accurately as possible in humans, the consequences of embryonic androgenization independent of postnatal endocrine changes (which are medically corrected). This helps in assessing the consequences of embryonic androgenization on the behavior of girls who are normally raised as such. [See the work of Melissa Hines, including (Hines & Kaufman, 1994; Brown et al., 2002b; Hines et al., 2003; Hines et al., 2004).] I shall return to this topic.

The Treatment of High-Risk Pregnancies by DES or Progestagen

There are also populations of girls whose mothers, during pregnancy, were exposed for medical reasons (treatment of risk of spontaneous abortion) to synthetic steroids such as diethylstilbestrol (DES) or acetate of medroxyprogesterone. It was realized afterward that some of these treatments were associated with masculinization of the reproductive function and behavior. These treatments were stopped as soon as doctors became aware of their consequences. People unfortunately exposed to this masculinizing action gave us another important source of information about the long-term behavioral effects of embryonic steroids.

SEXUAL DIFFERENTIATION OF BEHAVIOR

The physical effects of testosterone during embryonic development that I have just described leave, in my opinion, no doubt about the conclusion that in the human species, mechanisms of endocrine control of morphological sexual differentiation are identical in all respects to those reported in other mammals. Knowing that in rodents and monkeys these early physical effects of testosterone on sexual differentiation are accompanied by the sexual differentiation of many aspects of behavior, it is natural to ask whether human behaviors are also irreversibly affected by embryonic exposure to testosterone in young males (and its absence in the female embryo). The answer to this question is much more difficult because, although the morphology develops under the influence of hormones quite independently of external conditions, behavior is strongly influenced by interactions with parents, siblings, and all social relationships of young children. Influences that are not the same for babies of either sex (Hefez, 2007) will deeply affect the development of behavior. It is therefore very difficult to find during the child's development (and even more in the adult's) clear traces of a possible prenatal endocrine influence on the expression of behavioral traits. Even though absolute proof of the existence of such effects is lacking, some observations and clinical studies nonetheless suggest their presence.

A number of behavioral differences exist between men and women. Many of these differences have a rather limited magnitude (see Chapter 5), however, and seem to result mainly from the differential education of boys and girls. Others have a much greater magnitude and relate in particular to sexual orientation and sexual identity, two behavioral characteristics for which 90–99% of the population shows a marked sex difference closely correlated to the biological sex. The second part of this book is mainly devoted to the analysis of various arguments that strongly suggest that sexual orientation is determined by biological factors acting predominantly during the embryonic period.

Before addressing these arguments, it is important to ask whether steroids have organizing effects on behavior in humans and animals. In other words, does the hormonal milieu, in addition to determining genital form, influence the organization of behavior in a more masculine or feminine way? Given the impossibility for ethical reasons of implementing any type of experimentation on the subject, it is only through the analysis of clinical cases that we can try to answer this question. Moreover, because behavior is strongly influenced by education and social influences, we can hope to find a trace of an interpretable embryonic hormonal influence only in clinical cases where this hormonal influence is acting against the standards imposed by education.

For example, individuals affected by the syndrome of androgen insensitivity (AIS) teach us very little about the possible role of hormones in the differentiation of behavior. These individuals, with male sex chromosome (XY), have testes that secrete testosterone, but the steroid cannot act due to a mutation in the androgen receptor. Therefore they are born with female genitalia but are also raised as girls. They thus assume as adults the sexual orientation and gender identity of women, but it is impossible to know whether this is due to their education as a girl or the lack of effect of testosterone in the male embryo. These cases do demonstrate that the sex chromosomes are not very important as such: XY individuals may well develop a female phenotype. It is the hormonal action in the embryo that is critical for determining the phenotype at birth. Whether female behavioral traits observed in adulthood are the direct consequence of this embryonic hormonal action or a byproduct of the education of these subjects raised as girls remains impossible to ascertain.

Girls with the syndrome of Congenital Adrenal Hyperplasia (CAH) are, from this point of view, much more interesting and have therefore been the subject of many behavioral studies. Females with CAH were indeed exposed in utero to a hormonal milieu typical of the male (presence of large quantities of androgens of adrenal origin) but are generally raised as girls after postnatal surgical correction of their external genitals. If embryonic androgens affect the differentiation of sexual behavior, it could be expected that these girls would be to some extent behaviorally masculinized. And that is indeed what has been observed in several studies (Hines, 2003; Hines et al., 2003; Hines et al., 2004). The author of these studies has summarized the results in a book for the general public (Hines, 2004).

A classic behavioral difference between boys and girls concerns the type of games that they choose freely in a controlled test situation. If we introduce individual boys or girls in a room containing various types of toys, the girls spontaneously chose dolls while boys prefer to take cars or trains. Spontaneous games of boys are also more violent than in girls. One might think that this sex difference in children's behavior is entirely cultural and driven solely by the differential treatment of children by parents and society. In fact, it is not. It was demonstrated that these spontaneous toy choices are clearly masculinized in CAH in girls who have been exposed to abnormally high androgen levels during their life in utero but not during the postnatal period (thanks to medical treatment). In addition, play of CAH girls is more violent than in control girls not affected by prenatal androgenization (Figure 6.4) (Berenbaum & Snyder, 1995; Nordenstrom et al., 2002).

An interesting finding is that an offer of the same selection of toys to young vervet monkeys (*Cercopithecus aethiops sabaeus*) produces the same choice differences between sexes as found in humans: males are more interested in cars or balls whereas females are more interested in dolls (Figure 6.5a) (Alexander & Hines, 2002; Hassett et al., 2008).

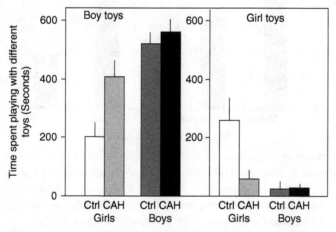

Figure 6.4 The type of toy used predominantly by boys and girls is sexually differentiated and influenced by the embryonic hormonal environment. Boys spend more time with toys such as cars or buildings tools (Boys Games), and girls with dolls, doll clothes, and kitchen utensils (Girls Toys). These preferences are significantly masculinized (increased time spent with the boys' toys) and defeminized (decrease of the time spent with the girls' toys) in CAH girls. The boys already have a lot of testosterone and their preference is not affected by additional testosterone related to CAH status. The results of the four types of subjects are represented by columns in which the intensity of gray is proportional to the concentration of testosterone supposed to have been present during embryonic life (according to Berenbaum & Snyder, 1995).

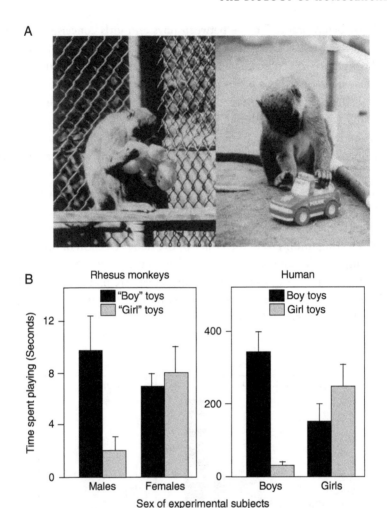

Figure 6.5 Young monkeys show the same preferences for different types of toys as human children. A. Photographs showing the play of young vervet monkeys with a doll (left) or a car (right). (Reproduced from Alexander & Hines, 2002, with permission.) B. Sex difference in time spent playing with boy or girl toys in rhesus monkeys or in humans (redrawn from Hassett et al., 2008; Berenbaum & Hines, 1992).

Recent experiments have now confirmed this result in another species of monkey, the rhesus (*Macaca mulatta*). Young males received toys classically considered in humans to be preferred by boys or girls: wheeled toys or stuffed animals, respectively. Toys with wheels were used far more frequently by rhesus males than by females, while young monkeys of both sexes played more or less equally with stuffed animals (Figure 6.5.b) (Alexander & Hines, 2002; Hassett et al., 2008). The comparison with the human data is striking. We also note that in this study, in the rhesus as in humans, the sex difference of use of toys for boys (cars) is much larger than the difference in the use of toys for girls (dolls, stuffed animals).

One might ask why monkeys differentially use toys that are obviously not of direct significance for them (cars or trains). The answer to this question should probably be sought in the properties of toys studied. Toys with wheels can, for example, allow games that are more active and could be preferred by males, given their propensity to engage in these types of games [see Williams & Pleil (2008) for a more detailed discussion on this subject]. These data suggest that sexually differentiated preferences for characteristics of objects (color, shape, movement) emerged very early in the lineage leading to human evolution. They may have been selected by evolutionary pressures related to the differential roles played by men and women and still be operant in the determinism of the choice of toys shown by small children.

The notion that these preferences are imposed only by society is contradicted by these observations. First, the monkeys had never been able to interact with the toys before the test, so it is impossible that education played a role. In addition, the CAH girls, although raised as girls, show preferences more or less masculinized for games that seem consistent with the hormonal milieu to which they were exposed in utero. The preferences observed are, instead, related to the general nature of the objects (e.g., preferences of boys and male monkeys for moving objects with wheels and more active games) (Hines & Alexander, 2008; Williams & Pleil, 2008) At the proximal level, these preferences appear to be controlled, at least in part, by the degree of in utero exposure to testosterone, as suggested by the study of CAH girls.

A study in Japan suggests, moreover, that there are sex differences in the types of drawings made voluntarily by children and that these drawings are masculinized in females affected by the CAH syndrome (Iijima et al., 2001). If we provide young children, five to six years old, with a set of colored pencils, boys on average tend to draw mechanical or moving objects with dark or cold colors (blue, green), while girls prefer drawing human beings (especially girls and women), flowers, or butterflies with warm colors (yellow, red). The drawings of boys are also more often drawings of objects seen from above, while girls tend to align objects at ground level. An analysis of drawings made by girls affected by the CAH syndrome has shown that their drawings did not have the usual female characteristics but were heavily masculinized and included all the features normally observed in the drawings of boys. Again, these observations strongly suggest that the embryonic hormonal environment plays a role in organizing this aspect of behavior. It should be noted that during early childhood (from more or less a year of age until the approach of puberty), levels of circulating testosterone are the same in boys and girls. Any influence of testosterone thus can only be a long-term influence of hormonal differences that were experienced during embryonic life.

The potential influence of the embryonic environment (masculinization) is contra to the type of education received (as a girl). It is thus logical to assume that the observed behavioral masculinization in CAH girls is due to their pre-natal exposure to abnormally high levels of androgens. In most cases, these girls are not completely masculine, and this aspect of their personality undoubtedly reflects the postnatal influence of parental and social environment. The influ-ence of education cannot be denied in humans (it is already clear in animals), but these clinical cases suggest very strongly that the influences on the behavior of the embryonic hormonal milieu that have been described in animals also exist in humans. Based on the principle of the unity of life and evolution of animal lineages, why would be otherwise?

Finally, the progress in psychological methods used to analyze the behavior of young children now allows us to test their response to various stimuli from an early age on, even during their first days of life, before any influence of edu-cation can take place. These studies show that very interesting sex differences in behavior are already present at that stage. In one study, British researchers from the laboratory of Simon Baron-Cohen filmed more than 100 babies, only one day old, while they were in the clinic being subjected to psychological tests. During these tests, the researchers showed an image of one of the researchers (JC), at a distance of 20 cm, in which she adopted a positive emotional expres-sion while remaining silent, or the image of a moving object (ball suspended from a 1 m stick) matched precisely for five aspects of the figure: color, size, shape, contrast, and tridimensional aspect (a small ball of 3 cm was attached in the middle of a mobile object at the same place as the nose). The mobile object was moved mechanically over the child's head at the same distance of 20 cm. All elements of the face of JC were present on the mobile, but completely mixed so that the presence of a human figure was no longer recognizable (Figure 6.6). To preserve the neutrality of the experimenters, researchers were not notified of the sex of the baby before the end of the tests and their analysis.

These studies have shown, quite surprisingly, that there is a significant differ-ence between boys and girls in their response to both visual stimuli (Connellan et al., 2000). The girls looked longer at the human face, but the boys looked more at the mobile. This difference at birth recalls another difference observed throughout the duration of life: on average, women interact more socially than men via social smiles and by maintaining direct eye contact. Although aspects of the methodology used in these studies have been criticized and its potential impact on adult sex differences has been questioned (Barres, 2010; Fine, 2010), the fact that such a sex difference has been observed at birth suggests the existence of a biological difference related to prenatal factors. In addition,

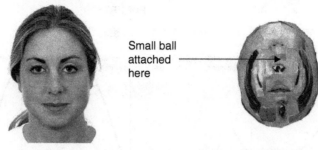

Face of researcher (JC)   Mobile object

Figure 6.6 Photograph of the stimuli used in the study of the gaze of one-day-old babies (reprinted from Connellan et al., 2000 with permission).

other studies of the group of Simon Baron-Cohen have shown that the amount of eye contact with parents of 12-month-old children was inversely correlated to the concentration of embryonic testosterone measured by amniocentesis between 14 and 21 weeks of gestation (Lutchmaya et al., 2002). There are therefore good reasons to believe that embryonic testosterone could be one of the factors responsible for individual and sex differences that affect certain aspects of social relationships (refer to the excellent popular books by Simon Baron-Cohen on the subject (Baron-Cohen, 2004; Baron-Cohen, 2006)).

THE MULTIPLE PEAKS OF TESTOSTERONE DURING DEVELOPMENT: POSSIBLE CONSEQUENCES FOR PHYSICAL AND BEHAVIORAL DIFFERENTIATION

An extremely important fact to mention is that during embryonic development of a normal male embryo and its postnatal life, testosterone is not secreted in high concentrations on a continuous basis (Figure 6.7).

In male embryos, an early peak of concentration in early gestation is responsible for morphological differentiation, followed by a period of slightly lower concentration that covers the second and third trimesters of pregnancy. These peaks do not occur in the female embryo. After a large peak immediately after birth, the secretion of testosterone is very low throughout infancy and will show a significant increase at puberty. At this point, it will trigger the final maturation of genital organs, spermatogenesis, and development of pubic hair. This period also corresponds to the onset of behavioral sexual activity.

It is firmly established that the differentiation of the genital structures of the human embryo takes place during the first two months of gestation, whereas the brain develops and differentiates during the second half of pregnancy. Thus, if an event were to alter the endocrine profile between these two periods, it is

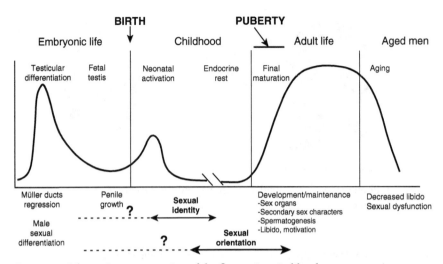

Figure 6.7 Schematic representation of the fluctuations in blood testosterone in men.

conceivable that the newborn may have a genital form (determined early in gestation) that does not correspond completely with some traits of his personality, such as his gender identity or sexual orientation, which are determined much later.

It therefore seems possible that an individual who has experienced "normal" conditions during the first part of his or her embryonic development has genital structures of one sex but that, subsequently, hormonal changes occur and may change his or her gender identity (transsexual) or sexual orientation (homosexual). These characteristics of an individual are firmly established in early childhood. The development of sexual orientation, however, does not become evident until later in life (puberty). Various clinical and epidemiological data suggest that sexual differentiation of these two characteristics could begin during the second half of embryonic life (Swaab, 2007).

The presence or absence of testosterone at different critical periods during development is not the only factor that can potentially generate discordance between the genetic and gonadal sex of an individual, on the one hand, and some of his or her behavioral characteristics, on another hand. To exert its actions, testosterone must be transformed into active metabolites (estradiol, DHT) that must bind to proper intracellular receptors and activate a cascade of biochemical events that will eventually lead to the biological response. Localized changes in any aspect of this reaction chain can therefore produce discordance between the actions of the steroids at two loci. The profile of plasma testosterone concentrations could thus be perfectly normal in a male subject, but local changes in testosterone action in the brain could prevent the full spectrum of steroid action in this structure, resulting in discordant behavioral features. I shall return to these ideas in the sections devoted specifically to homosexuality (see Chapter 8).

SEXUAL DIFFERENTIATION OF THE BRAIN

A number of differences between the sexes have been identified in the human brain (Chapter 5). These differences relate to the size of a sexually dimorphic nucleus of preoptic area (SDN-POA) (Swaab & Fliers, 1985; Allen et al., 1989; LeVay, 1991), the bed nucleus of the stria terminalis (BST) (Zhou et al., 1995; Chung et al., 2002), and thick bundles of fibers connecting the left and right sides of the brain (de Lacoste-Utamsing & Holloway, 1982) (the anterior commissure and the corpus callosum) [see (Dubb et al., 2003; Tuncer et al., 2005; Ozdemir et al., 2007) for a potential challenge of this difference]. Difficulties in obtaining human brains for histological analysis, combined with the relative scarcity of endocrine diseases disrupting sexual differentiation, explain why, to date, no study has specifically analyzed the contribution of sex steroids in embryonic development on sex differences observed in the nervous system.

Two studies, however, have evaluated the postnatal ontogenesis of sex differences that affect the volume of the sexually dimorphic nucleus of preoptic area and the bed nucleus of the stria terminalis and have shown that these structures are not fully differentiated at birth. For example, the SDN-POA, as described by Swaab and collaborators, at birth only contains 20% of the cells that it contains at two to four years of age. This number of cells is believed to increase quickly and in the same way in boys and girls between birth and two to four years. Only after this period does a decrease in the number of neurons specifically affecting girls create a sex difference in volume (Swaab & Hofman, 1988). These critical events occur, therefore, in early childhood, when circulating levels of testosterone are the same in both sexes. Similarly, it was shown that the sex difference in volume affecting the bed nucleus of the stria terminalis is not present in children and is expressed only in adults (Chung et al., 2002).

Recall that in rats, the larger volume of the sexually dimorphic nucleus of the preoptic area is determined exclusively by the prenatal and perinatal effects of testosterone (Jacobson et al., 1981; Arnold & Gorski, 1984). This difference is determined entirely prenatally in sheep. It is important to note that, in rats as well, volumetric differences of the SDN are not necessarily present at birth (Jacobson et al., 1980). They continue to develop during the first weeks of life under the influence of increased neuronal death in females (Davis et al., 1995). It is likely that early hormonal action sets in motion a series of mechanisms that will continue to act during the postnatal prepubescent life in the absence of significant concentrations of testosterone. This situation is perhaps not so different from what happens in humans, and we have as yet no reason to believe that the difference in volume of the SDN-POA present in humans develops by mechanisms different from those described in rats or sheep. But we do not have any argument beyond evolutionary continuity to confirm the identity of these mechanisms.

Some authors (e.g. Vidal, 2007, p. 13) argue that the sexually dimorphic nucleus of the hypothalamus would be unable to control sexual orientation. C. Vidal announces a size of 50 microns of this sexually dimorphic nucleus in women and homosexuals and 100 microns in heterosexual men (cubic microns, I assume). Although small (between 0.05 mm^3 in homosexuals and 0.10 mm^3 in heterosexuals), the human SDN contains a significant number of neurons, approximately 1,800. It is generally accepted that each neuron in the human brain on average makes 100 to 1,000 connections with other neurons. This means that the SDN is directly connected to a number of neurons ranging between 18,000 and 180,000, themselves part of a network that is branching in an exponential manner. Such a network is capable, I believe, of managing complex information. Excluding a priori that it could be a significant part of the mechanisms that control sexual orientation is not based on any rational argument, even if the author of this book was trained as a neurobiologist and director of research at the Pasteur Institute. The denial of the role of the brain is here based on a priori excluding the idea that there may be significant differences between the male and female brains. If the ultimate goal of this claim is laudable (fight against sex discrimination), the means are not scientifically acceptable.

7

The Effects of Sex Steroids in Humans

Activating Effects

FORMS AND FUNCTIONS

There are numerous effects of sex steroids (androgens, estrogens, and progesta-gens) during the postnatal life in man and woman. These effects are impossible to ignore and widely known to the general public. At puberty, because of the significant increase in circulating testosterone concentrations in young males, the penis increases in size and the testes grow larger and start producing sperm. In parallel, muscles develop, pubic and armpit hair appears, and the tone of voice drops (deeper voice) due to the thickening of the vocal cords. All these effects are, entirely or in part, caused by testosterone. If testosterone is not pres-ent due to a failure of testicular function or following an accidental or voluntary castration (e.g., Italian castrati, eunuchs for harems), none of this maturation related to puberty will occur.

From a theoretical point of view, it should be noted that many of these effects are irreversible. Some researchers thus consider puberty to be a second phase of organization of physical form and function that complements the sexual dif-ferentiation that occurs during the months before and after birth (Sisk & Zehr, 2005; Ahmed et al., 2008).

In young females, puberty is marked by the onset of ovarian activity, which, for the next 30 to 40 years, produces estrogen and progesterone in a cyclical fashion in association with the cycle of ovulation and menstruation. Puberty also brings the appearance of pubic hair and (later) armpit hair, a development of the lips of the vulva, and a deepening and thickening of the walls of the vagina. It is also the time when breasts are developing that in a few years will reach their adult size. Ovarian estrogens are largely responsible for these changes in the girl during puberty, but androgens secreted by the adrenal glands also play a particular role in the development of the hair. If for any reason ovarian activity and menstruation do not appear, the changes of form just described will not be observed.

The role of androgens in the development of hair in women (and men, of course) is also well established by the fact that the alterations of adrenal activity associated with increased production of androgens always result in an increased hairiness affecting the same area, the face ("bearded woman"). During menopause, which corresponds to the cessation of ovarian activity, there is also often a slight increase in the secretion of androgens by the adrenal glands, often accompanied by a slight development of facial hair (beard and mustache).

BEHAVIOR

If the reality of the effects of sex steroids on the morphology (including genital) and the physiology of reproduction does not appear to be contested, there is in contrast a widespread reluctance to accept the idea that sex steroids could play a role in control of behavior in general and sexual behavior in particular. This resistance is particularly important in Latin societies. For instance, in *Men and Women: Do We Have the Same Brain?* Catherine Vidal wrote, "In animals, the action of hormones on the brain induces mating behavior and mating periods are associated with ovulation of the female. Sexuality and reproduction go hand in hand. In contrast the human being escapes this determinism" (Vidal, 2007). There is, in my opinion, no statement more false than her last sentence.

Human sexual behavior is very complex, and its control involves multiple cognitive aspects (experience, perception of social expectations of the environment, individual preferences, social conventions, varied religious and philosophical influences, etc.), the importance of which relates to the major development of the cerebral cortex that characterizes our species. Accordingly, the mere presence of testosterone in the blood and brain of a man and of estradiol in a woman will not automatically lead them to have sex (mating) within minutes of their first meeting. It is also not the case in animals. The specific studies conducted in particular in rats and mice are showing the influence of multiple variables on sexual behavior in these species, such as prior experience, learning, individual preferences, and the effect of an audience on the social behavior achieved. Only in the study of instinctive reactions in invertebrates such as insects do we find to some degree the automatic causal reactions between hormones and behavior that is erroneously considered as being typical of animal sexuality.

The decision to engage in sex with a sexual partner in the human species does not depend solely on circulating testosterone levels of men and estradiol in women, but it will certainly be influenced by these hormonal factors in a more or less direct manner (see below). Sexual motivation in humans remains under hormonal control even if it is partially emancipated, as is partly the case in the animal lineage in parallel with the development of the brain and especially of the cortex. If sexual motivation were entirely the result of learning and a social construction, we should then wonder why no society has ever managed to put its expectations in line with the behavior of individuals. Sex outside marriage is discouraged or prohibited, for example, by many human societies. In some cases, adultery is still punishable by death, sometimes by methods that could be very discouraging, such as lapidation (stoning). The fact is, however, that sex outside marriage remains present even in these societies.

I believe that sexual motivation in humans and animals is essentially the result of the action of sex steroids on the brain and in particular on preoptic, hypothalamic, and limbic (amygdala) regions. Philosophical or social contingencies have an important role in determining whether the individual will adopt a behavior in agreement with this motivation. Religious or social prohibitions can, for example, prevent an individual from having an extra-marital relationship. Here cortical activity takes precedence over the impulse originating in hypothalamic or limbic areas, *but the motivation remains*. This cannot be emphasized too strongly! Innumerable literary works examine the conflict between the sex drive and social prohibitions consciously managed by the cortex. This motivation is also modulated by many other factors (e.g., lack of sexual desire in a situation of stress), but the main determinant remains hormones in humans and animals. Many arguments support this thesis.

EVOLUTIONARY ARGUMENT

The brain regions that are known to control sexual behavior in rodents and primates have changed very little from a physical or neurochemical point of view between mammals and humans. Humans possess almost all the nuclei (clusters of neurons) of the preoptic area, hypothalamus, and limbic systems that control sexual behavior in the rat brain. In addition to this anatomical consistency, the same neurotransmitters as in animals and steroid hormone receptors (androgen and estrogen receptors) that have been characterized in other vertebrates are also found in these regions of the human brain. The distribution of these receptors is very consistent from fish to mammals (Kelley & Pfaff, 1978; Morrell & Pfaff, 1978), and man is no exception (Kruijver et al., 2001; Kruijver et al., 2002; 2003). The cellular and neurochemical "machinery" underlying the expression of sexual behavior in vertebrates is therefore intact in humans. Its persistence indicates that there are evolutionary pressures that maintain it in place and function. If, as I claim here, these neural circuits control sexual motivation under the influence of ovarian and testicular steroids, the nature of this selective pressure becomes immediately obvious.

TEMPORAL AND INDIVIDUAL CORRELATIONS

The sex steroids are not present in constant quantities throughout life. If they play a significant role in the control of sexual activity, one would expect a positive correlation between changes in the time of the concentrations of steroids and frequency of sexual activity. This is indeed what has been observed in many studies of both men and women.

Measurement of the blood levels of testosterone of a large number of men during their lifetime yields a series of reproducible values that are positioned on a generally inverted U-curve (see Chapter 6, Figure 6.7). The ascending phase of this curve corresponds precisely to the puberty and onset of sexual activity. The peak of this curve is between 20 and 60 years and corresponds to the maximum of sexual activity in humans. Then begins a gradual decrease of circulating levels of steroid associated with the well-documented decline in sexual activity with age (Vermeulen et al., 1972). There is wide individual variation around this mean curve, and it would be ridiculous to suggest that changes in concentration of steroid alone explain the distribution of sexual activity during the life of man. The beginning and end of this activity, however, are linked quite closely to changes in blood concentration.

The relationship between hormones and behavior can also be greatly strengthened by studying individual variations in periods of instability. Various researchers have analyzed the relationship between increased blood levels of testosterone at the time of puberty and the appearance of male sexual behavior. Since a continuous and accurate record of this behavior is impossible, researchers have relied on more indirect, rough measures, such as the age of first sexual relationship or the likelihood of having had sex at a given age. Even with measures this imprecise, a very strong connection appears between hormone and behavior. Figure 7.1 illustrates the relationship between salivary testosterone (salivary concentrations are a fairly accurate reflection of blood levels), expressed as deviations from the average values (mean plus or minus one, two or three standard deviations, a measure of variability), and the probability at a given age that a boy has already had sex. There is an excellent correlation between these two measures, suggesting that testosterone levels higher than average are associated with greater sexual activity (Halpern et al., 1998).

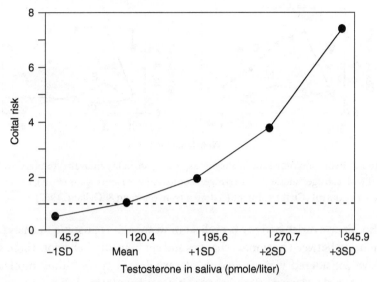

Figure 7.1 Relationship between the concentration of testosterone in saliva and the probability of occurrence of complete sexual (coital) behavior in adolescents (age 12–13 years at baseline). Saliva samples were collected at regular intervals over a period of two years during which the subjects filled out questionnaires about their weekly sexual activity. The average risk of coital sexual behavior is adjusted to 1 for average values of testosterone (120.4 pmol/l). It increases in an exponential manner when concentrations of testosterone increased by 1, 2, or 3 standard deviations (SD) above average (redrawn from Halpern et al. 1998).

This type of relationship has been observed both in transversal studies of a large number of individuals of the same age (Udry et al., 1985) and in longitudinal studies that followed a smaller number of subjects during their development (Halpern et al., 1998). These relationships also appear to be independent of the societies and cultures in which the boys live. Similar correlations between testosterone levels and age at first sexual relationship have recently been identified in a population in Zimbabwe (Campbell et al., 2005).

In women, a similar relationship between the individual values of blood concentrations of testosterone and the onset of sexual activity has been identified by the same methods (Halpern et al., 1997). Testosterone appears to be involved also in the activation of sexual motivation in women; this hormone is prescribed in combination with estrogen to increase sexual desire in women whose ovaries have been removed for medical reasons (Figure 7.2). Controlled studies demonstrated an increase in sexual desire, sexual fantasies, and sexual arousal in response to treatment with androgens combined with estrogens. In contrast, estrogens alone had no effect (Sherwin & Gelfand, 1987).

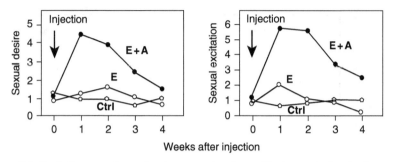

Figure 7.2 Evolution over time of various aspects of sexuality in ovariectomized women treated with estrogen alone (E) or estrogen combined with androgens (E+A), or receiving a control (Ctrl) treatment (redrawn from Sherwin & Gelfand 1987).

Also, since ovarian activity is cyclical in women, it is possible to analyze the relationship between hormonal changes and spontaneous behavior. These studies have considered various aspects of sexual activity, including motivation (desire) but also sexual attractiveness. It must be admitted that many results in this context have proved to be difficult to reproduce or not reproducible. Some studies have reported the existence of a peak of sexual activity in women at the time of ovulation [for details see LeVay & Valente (2006) p. 142]. This peak could represent a remnant of estrus in animals. In many species, sexual activity of the female is indeed restricted to the periovulatory period. Peaks of activity, however, have also been reported in humans at other times of the cycle (premenstrual period) and have no obvious functional or evolutionary interpretation. These periovulatory peaks, when observed, are probably the result of hormonal changes associated with the cycle, because some studies indicate that these behavioral changes are not observed in women who undergo hormonal contraception that makes their hormonal environment constant during most of the ovarian cycle.

The reasons underlying the variability of the results of these studies are not always identified but include the possibility of inadequate characterization of the hormonal status of women studied (e.g., a single dose of blood unrepresentative of the average hormonal state because of rapid fluctuations of hormone levels, hormonal status inferred from the stage of the menstrual cycle but not confirmed by direct measurements of plasma levels), the obscuring of the correlation of hormone-influenced behavior by nonhormonal factors (daily problems interfering with sexual desire, unrecognized medical problems, etc.), or vague or biased recording of actual sexual activity.

Even if better-controlled studies confirm the presence of a periovulatory peak of sexual activity among women, the interpretation of this peak will remain difficult because it could result equally from either an increase in the sexual motivation of the women or an increase in their attractiveness. Studies have attempted to isolate these two interpretations by documenting (with questionnaires), in stable couples, the frequency of sexual activity that was initiated by the woman (and supposedly related to her motivation) or initiated by the man (reflecting hormone-related changes in the woman's attractiveness), but it appears that the variability in these studies makes it impossible to draw reproducible conclusions.

In a recent study, U.S. researchers adopted a very creative protocol to quantify potential changes during the menstrual cycle of attractiveness of a group of women in a situation that would minimize uncontrolled extraneous variables (Miller et al., 2007). They recorded the tips earned by seminude (topless) women dancing in nightclubs ("lap dancers") and correlated the tips with the stage of the women's menstrual cycle. These women dance on a podium several times each evening to an audience, but under these conditions they will collect only small tips. During the remainder of the evening, they walk in the room and offer to "dance" on the laps of customers during a period of about 3 minutes. During this activity they usually receive a larger tip, which often varies between $10 and $20 U.S. but is not fixed by any rule. These "dances" typically involve intensive rhythmic contacts between the pelvic region of women and the penis of the man, who is dressed and cannot touch the dancer with his hands. They represent the most intense form of paid sexual interaction that is permitted by U.S. law. Customers are able to assess the attractiveness of the dancers through very intimate verbal, visual, tactile, and olfactory sexual contacts. This type of situation is likely to more accurately evaluate attractiveness than in situations that were used previously and were based on the evaluation of photos or the voice of individuals tested.

The researchers asked the dancers to record the total amount of their earnings in the night club and their working time each day for 60 days. They were also to indicate the dates of their menstruations. Data from 18 women with regular menstrual cycles (28–30 days) were finally analyzed. Seven of them were using hormonal contraception, the other 11 did not use contraception and had not used it during the three months preceding the study. As indicated in Figure 7.3, gratuities earned by women during their fertile period (periovulatory) were twice as high as what they earned in luteal phase (the part of the menstrual cycle following ovulation) or during menstruation. These variations in gains were significant and were not observed in women using the contraceptive pill, which equalizes the circulating hormone concentrations during most of the cycle.

These data support the idea that sexual attractiveness in women varies during the ovarian cycle and that these variations in attractiveness are due to fluctuations associated with the hormonal cycle. Further research should be undertaken to test the reproducibility of these findings and identify the nature of signals that modulate attractiveness (verbal, visual, or olfactory).

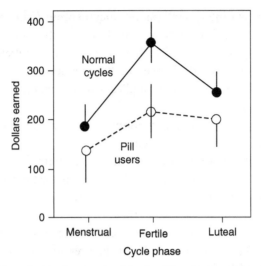

Figure 7.3 Variations during the menstrual cycle of female attractiveness assessed indirectly by the dollar amount of tips obtained by seminude dancers in cabaret. A peak gain is observed in ovulatory phase (fertile) compared to menstrual and luteal phases. This temporal variation is not present in women using an oral contraceptive and who therefore have a constant level of estrogen and progesterone during the cycle (redrawn from Miller et al. 2007).

THE ANALYSIS AND TREATMENT OF CLINICAL CASES

Numerous clinical studies have been conducted on different types of patients suffering from various sexual problems. These studies reinforce the notion that male sexual activity is controlled at least partly by testosterone. For example, there are patients with pathologically low development of the testes, which therefore produce abnormally low testosterone concentrations (hypogonadism). Many of these subjects have a low sexual activity associated with a low frequency of nocturnal erections, episodes of masturbation, and orgasms. Julian Davidson showed that treatment of these subjects by a single injection with a form of testosterone that is released gradually into the blood (testosterone enanthate) increases all the measures of sexual activity included in this study, proportional to the dosage, while restoring more normal blood levels of testosterone (Davidson et al., 1979).

Many similar studies have since confirmed this conclusion, including a blind clinical study (the subjects did not know which treatment was administered), again on hypogonadic men, that showed that after two years of treatment with testosterone, over 80% of subjects considered that their libido had improved, while less than 10% held this view in the control group (Hajjar et al., 1997) (Figure 7.4).

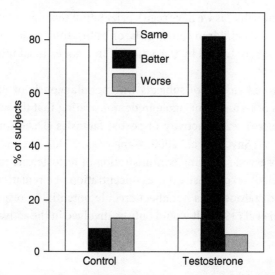

Figure 7.4 Percentage of male subjects suffering from hypogonadism in which sex life had improved, deteriorated, or remained the same after two years of treatment with testosterone or a control treatment (according to Hajjar et al. 1997).

The role of testosterone has also been demonstrated in initially normal patients in a very elegant study conducted at the Veterans Administration Medical Center in Seattle. For 6 weeks, male volunteers were treated with an antagonist of GnRH (gonadotrophin releasing hormone or gonadoliberin). This hormone, normally produced by the hypothalamus, stimulates the synthesis of the two gonadotropic hormones (LH and FSH) in the pituitary gland, which in turn act on the testes to produce secretion of testosterone. In the chronic presence of an antagonist (receptor blocker) of GnRH, levels of circulating testosterone drop rapidly. The treated subjects observed a strong parallel decrease of their interest in sex. They had fewer sexual fantasies, masturbated less often, and the frequency of sex decreased. A fraction of these subjects were simultaneously treated with testosterone in sufficient quantity to maintain their circulating concentrations at normal physiological levels, and they accordingly experienced no decrease in sexual motivation (Bagatell et al., 1994).

There is also a biomedical literature that indicates that the treatment of sexual offenders by androgen antagonists or GnRH antagonists that suppress either the action or the secretion of testosterone diminishes the sex drive. However, in many of these studies, the decrease of sexual motivation was a condition for release from jail of the offenders. The objectivity of their statements about their sexual motivation may therefore be questioned, and the value of the conclusions drawn from these studies is questionable. It is also interesting to note that even if the sexual motivation of these offenders is decreased (which is questionable, as we have seen), orientation remains the same and they are still attracted by children (boys, girls, or both), thus indicating that sexual orientation is not controlled by the action of hormones in adulthood, as I discuss in Chapter 8.

Nevertheless, all studies of subjects with spontaneously or experimentally very low levels of testosterone agree in demonstrating that the addition of testosterone increases sexual activity or sexual fantasies (Davidson et al., 1979; Hajjar et al., 1997; Snyder et al., 2000; Wang et al., 2000). In contrast, improvement is not observed following administration of testosterone to subjects suffering from lack of sexual desire if the concentration of circulating testosterone is normal. Testosterone does not affect erectile potential in response to erotic stimuli (Carani et al., 1992). It would only be involved in the activation of sexual motivation.

8

Sex Differences Suggest Homosexuality Is an Endocrine Phenomenon

Two major types of biological nonexclusive explanations have been advanced to explain homosexual sexual behavior. Either it is controlled by hormonal factors that are known to play a role in the control of animal behavior and its sexual orientation, or it depends on genetic factors that work independently of hormones or by altering their production or action. I consider in this chapter and in Chapter 9 arguments that suggest the existence of hormonal control mechanisms of homosexuality.

HORMONES ARE "NORMAL" IN ADULT HOMOSEXUALS: NO DIFFERENCE IN ACTIVATION

Knowing that sex steroids play a key role in the activation of sexual behavior in animals and in humans, researchers have logically thought that disturbances in circulating concentrations of these hormones could be involved in the control of homosexuality. In animals and to some extent in humans, testosterone activates the male-typical sexual behavior, and estradiol combined with progesterone activates female-typical sexual behavior. One could imagine that the presence of excessive levels of estradiol in some men is responsible for their sexual attraction to other men (a female characteristic) and that, vice versa, high concentrations of testosterone induce female sexual attraction toward other women (a feature normally observed in men). This old theory has been regarded as plausible by some scientists, and it still enjoys a certain popularity in the public, but it is obviously inconsistent with animal studies that have established that the type of behavior produced by males or females is not conditioned by the type of hormones to which they are exposed in adulthood but rather by the sex of their brain, which is determined during ontogenesis (organizing effects of sex steroids, see Chapter 3).

Since accurate and reproducible assays of sex steroids became available during the 1960s and 1970s, many studies have tested this hypothesis by comparing the concentrations of circulating sex steroids in men and women in relation to their sexual orientation. The result of this work is very clear: no hormonal difference seems to exist between homosexual or heterosexual males or between homosexual or heterosexual women (Meyer-Bahlburg, 1984). Sexual orientation is not linked in humans to an inadequate activation by sex steroids considered typical of their sex. Gay men have levels of circulating testosterone that are perfectly normal, and the same applies for the concentrations of estradiol and progesterone in homosexual women. This conclusion is by no means surprising in light of the knowledge accumulated in animal studies. There used to be a confusion between the type of behavior patterns expressed by the animal (male-typical or female-typical sexual performance) and its orientation (toward a same-sex or opposite-sex partner). When this distinction was clearly established, it became clear that sexual orientation is not affected by treatment with sex steroids in adulthood. Only lesions of the preoptic area or hormonal manipulations made during ontogeny (embryonic or early postnatal) can achieve this goal (Chapter 4). Furthermore, the circulating testosterone levels are not altered in homosexual sheep as compared to subjects with a heterosexual orientation. It is therefore not surprising that the circulating hormone levels are perfectly normal among gay men and women. This also explains why attempts to change sexual orientation through hormone treatments have always failed.

CORRELATES OF HOMOSEXUALITY THAT SUGGEST
PRENATAL HORMONAL DETERMINISM

Knowing that in animals sexual differentiation of reproductive behavior and of sexual orientation is controlled by the action of embryonic steroids, researchers began looking at the logical consequences. Among the first to do so was endocrinologist Günter Dörner, who proposed a theory of homosexuality based on hormonal embryonic imprinting (Dörner, 1969). According to this theory, human fetuses destined to become gay in adulthood would experience an abnormal sexual differentiation due, for example, to exposure to abnormally low testosterone concentration in boys or a too high level of this hormone for girls or to a modified response of the brain to these hormones (see also Chapter 9).

Various arguments of a correlative nature suggest that sexual orientation in humans could be determined, at least in part, by the early hormonal imprinting (difference in the organization by steroids). The homosexual attraction in humans is the attraction normally present in a heterosexual woman (attraction to men) and vice versa. Homosexuality could easily be conceived, from a theoretical point of view, as the result of the sexual differentiation of this trait being reversed. Thus one can imagine that a lack of masculinization or incomplete masculinization of this behavioral characteristic results in adult men with a homosexual or bisexual orientation (a sexual orientation toward men, "normally" characteristic of females). Conversely, a female embryo's excessive exposure to androgens would result in an abnormal masculinization of the resulting behavioral trait in adulthood and in the male characteristic of a sexual attraction toward other women.

Knowing that the genital structures differentiate much earlier in embryonic life than the brain (see Chapter 6), it is conceivable that in a given individual, hormones can induce a "normal" development (corresponding to the genetic sex) of genital structures and that later during embryogenesis, hormonal changes can occur such that the differentiation of the brain and sexual orientation do not occur as expected. This model is perfectly consistent from the theoretical point of view and would be in complete agreement with animal studies that have been described previously.

For fairly obvious reasons, it is impossible or very difficult to know what hormonal milieu an adult was exposed to during embryonic life. Measures of the concentrations of circulating testosterone or estradiol in the embryo are associated with a significant risk (taking blood may cause an interruption of pregnancy), and this risk is taken only when required by serious medical reasons but in no case to make a scientific study, whatever its interest.

However, taking advantage of measurements made during amniocenteses prescribed for medical reasons, several years ago English researcher Simon Baron-Cohen begun analyzing the relationship between testosterone levels faced by the human embryo and various behavioral characteristics related mainly to social skills (what he calls the predisposition to empathy vs. systematization) of young children. Very interesting correlations have been found (Baron-Cohen, 2006). However, the number of subjects is limited and so far these studies have only looked into young children.

Extending such studies to homosexuality involves facing two issues. There is the very long latency (often exceeding 20 years) between the embryonic hormonal event supposed to induce homosexuality and its consequences, which are not seen until adulthood. There is also the limited frequency of homosexuality (2 to 8% of the population). It would be necessary to follow in detail the hormonal changes of a large number of randomly selected embryos, retain such data for over 20 years, find these subjects in adulthood, and obtain information on their sexual orientation (not always openly stated) in order to draw direct conclusions from this study. No researcher has yet had the ability to conduct such a long study, so this type of data does not exist.

We are therefore forced to rely on indirect evidence of what the hormonal embryonic milieu of homosexual individuals might have been. Many traits are irreversibly affected by embryonic hormones in animals and in humans. Researchers have thus been able to identify many characteristics that are different among men and women (see the next sections) as a result of a differential exposure of male and female embryos to embryonic sex steroid. Many studies have sought to evaluate these characteristics in a comparative manner in populations of homosexual and heterosexual subjects to determine whether homosexuals were exposed to atypical hormonal conditions during embryonic development. Many positive results have been gathered.

Homosexuality is not simply a different sexual orientation; it is accompanied by many changes. These changes usually concern characteristics that are sexually differentiated in the heterosexual population, related for example to the functioning of the inner ear and of specific parts of the brain. There is also a significant change in some cognitive abilities of individuals, including sexually differentiated aptitudes not related to sexuality, such as verbal skills or the ability to visualize three-dimensional space, not to mention differences in the length of bones and even in some brain structures. All the differences that were detected suggest the existence of hormonal differences in homosexual individuals during their infancy or embryonic life.

These studies have another significant interest. They indicate that homosexuality is not only a change in sexual orientation but is also reliably associated with physical (e.g., relative size of index and ring finger of the hand), functional (activity of the inner ear), and behavioral (various cognitive skills) differences unrelated to sexual behavior, though at the behavioral level the reproducibility of results seems lower and their interpretation more complex. These associations indicate in an indirect but fairly convincing manner that homosexuality is not a lifestyle choice to anywhere near the degree that most people believe it is. It is difficult to imagine how life choices could induce a change in the relative size of the fingers or a differential functioning of the inner ear. These differences obviously precede the appearance of homosexual orientation, and the most straightforward and plausible interpretation is that the same cause (probably hormonal) is responsible for all of them. I now describe in more detail these differences between homosexual and heterosexual individuals that are not directly related to sexual behavior.

COGNITIVE AND BEHAVIORAL DIFFERENCES
NOT DIRECTLY RELATED TO SEX

There are many differences in cognitive abilities between men and women. These differences often have rather limited amplitude (see Chapter 5), but many studies have shown that, on average, men tend to have better results than women in mathematical reasoning and in the performance of visual-spatial tasks. In contrast, women are better than men on tests measuring verbal ability, speed of calculation, the recognition of facial expressions, and memorizing the location of objects (Kiumura, 1999; Baron-Cohen, 2004).

Education clearly plays a major role in the genesis of these differences (Chapter 5) but there are data showing that the behavioral differences observed in adulthood result, at least in part, from prenatal differences in hormone concentrations between male and female embryos—that is, the differences partly result from the organizing effects of steroids (Collaer & Hines, 1995). The cognitive differences between men and women would be the result of biological differences and cultural differences that are likely to be mutually reinforcing, but the relative importance of these two types of effects remains to be determined [see Baron-Cohen (2004) for a more detailed discussion of this issue].

If we consider the possibility that homosexuality is due, at least in part, to an atypical embryonic hormonal milieu, it is then logical to ask whether the characteristics of cognitive functioning that are sexually differentiated (i.e., differ between men and women) are different as well in homosexuals compared to heterosexuals. Several studies have been devoted to this subject and have provided positive responses.

Tests for Which Men Are on Average Better than Women

VISUAL-SPATIAL TASKS
Several studies have shown that homosexual men have performances inferior to those of heterosexuals in the execution of many tasks, including visual-spatial mental rotation tasks, evaluation of the orientation of a straight line, and aiming at a specific target (Hall & Kimura, 1995; Neave et al., 1999; Rahman & Wilson, 2003b). Gay men generally have performances similar to those of women or intermediate between men and women. Some studies, however, have not shown such differences between homosexual and heterosexual males for some of these characteristics (Gladue et al., 1990; Tutle & Pillard, 1991).

Studies conducted in women, which according to this theory should identify masculinized performances in lesbians, have yielded results that are less clear. A recent study indicates that homosexual women perform mental rotations slightly better than heterosexual women, but the difference only affects the speed of execution of the task, not its accuracy (Rahman & Wilson, 2003b).

AGGRESSION

In general, men are more aggressive than women, and two separate studies have indicated that gay men are less physically aggressive than heterosexual men (Ellis et al., 1990). No difference in aggression has been identified between lesbians and heterosexual women (Gladue & Bailey, 1995). One can imagine that the basal level is very low, so a small increase can pass unnoticed.

Tests for Which Women Are on Average Better than Men

REMEMBERING THE LOCATION OF OBJECTS

A study based on a large number of subjects has shown that gay men localize objects more efficiently than heterosexuals, a finding that is consistent with this feature not having been fully masculinized (that is, increased to male levels by embryonic testosterone) in homosexuals. However, no difference was observed in this study between homosexual and heterosexual women (Rahman et al., 2003a).

VERBAL FLUENCY

A 1991 study indicated that homosexual men have a higher verbal performance than heterosexuals, a finding that conforms with the notion that they were not completely masculinized and therefore are more feminine from this point of view (McCormick & Witelson, 1991). Two subsequent studies have not been able to confirm this difference (Gladue et al., 1990). In addition, a recent analysis based on a large number of subjects reported that in verbal fluency tests, both gay men and gay women have performances that are atypical for their gender (Rahman et al., 2003a). Thus, in one of these tests, gay men were better than all other groups (heterosexual men and women regardless of their orientation). In another test, gay men and heterosexual women were better than lesbians and heterosexual men. These data indicate that for these features, gay men are more similar to women, whereas lesbians are more like men.

Feature Not Usually Differentiated: Manual Lateralization

Several studies have shown that both gay men and gay women tend not to be right-handed (instead, either left-handed or ambidextrous) significantly more frequently than heterosexual individuals (Lalumiere et al., 2000; Lippa, 2003b). This feature is not generally regarded as sexually differentiated in the heterosexual population, in which there are as many right-handed or left-handed or ambidextrous subjects among men as among women (Lippa, 2003b).

However, the existence of a predominant development of the right side of the body among men, whereas the left side would be favored in women, has been suggested (Baron-Cohen, 2004).

A recent meta-analysis of five independent studies also confirms the existence of a higher probability among homosexual men of not being right-handed (Blanchard & Lippa, 2007). This increased frequency of non–right-handedness is interesting from the point of view of the ontogenesis of homosexuality because the preferential use of one hand over the other is an individual trait observable before birth (Hepper et al., 1991), even if a reversal of lateralization is possible after a trauma, such as that associated with a difficult birth. The higher incidence of non–right-handedness among homosexuals of both sexes would be consistent with the idea of a prenatal determination of this orientation.

These differences in cognitive abilities or in lateralization related to homosexuality are, of course, consistent with the idea that an atypical embryonic hormonal milieu may have influenced the two types of variables in parallel. However, the hormonal contribution to these cognitive traits is probably limited (the role of the postnatal environment is important here), and many differences have a low reproducibility. These cognitive changes observed in homosexuals only moderately support the hormonal theory of homosexuality.

PERIPHERAL PHYSICAL DIFFERENCES

A good number of physical traits are also different between men and women and/or are known to be permanently influenced by embryonic hormones. Some of these traits are modified in homosexuals, thus suggesting again that they were exposed in utero to abnormally high or low concentrations of sex steroids. Two groups of reproducible studies on such characteristics are of interest, although not fully conclusive.

Index/Ring Finger Length Ratio

For most women, the index (finger 2 or D2) is almost as long as the ring finger (finger 4 or D4), so that the ratio of length D2:D4 is very close to 1 (0.973 on average). In males, the D2:D4 ratio is smaller (around 0.955) (see Figure 8.1).

This sex difference in the relative length of fingers probably reflects differences in the embryonic hormonal milieu (androgen concentrations higher in male fetuses than females) at the time of development and growth of the fingers. It is known that testosterone modulates the growth of long bones in the human embryo, as in other vertebrates. This notion is consistent with the fact that girls exposed to high androgen levels due to congenital hyperplasia of the adrenal glands (CAH, see Chapter 6) have a masculinized D2:D4 ratio, a lower

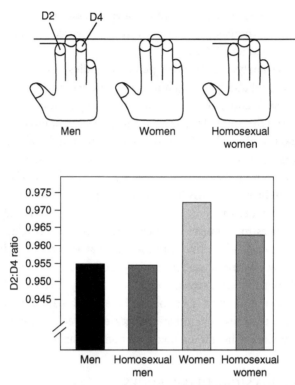

Figure 8.1 Ratio of lengths of the index (D2) and ring finger (D4) and sexual orientation. The ratio D2:D4 is higher in women than in men. It is close to the male level in homosexual women, thus suggesting they may have been exposed to abnormally high levels of testosterone during embryonic life. This ratio is not consistently changed in gay men as compared to heterosexual men.

ratio than in "normal" women (Brown et al., 2002b). A recent study also indicates that the D2:D4 ratio is higher in XY women affected by the complete androgen insensitivity syndrome (AIS) than in control XY males (Berenbaum et al., 2009). Moreover, this sex difference in the relative length of fingers is found in various animal species as well (Brown et al., 2002a; Romano et al., 2005) and is in animals significantly affected by early treatments with androgens (Lutchmaya et al., 2004; Romano et al., 2005; Manning et al., 2006). Together, these facts strongly suggest that the D2:D4 ratio is indeed affected by prenatal androgen levels [see Breedlove (2010) for a recent review], but it has been pointed out that the real world might actually be more complex than suggested by this simple conclusion. The ratio might be related more directly to the ratio of androgens to estrogens and might reflect a difference in adiposity rather than a true difference in finger lengths (Wallen, 2009).

Several independent groups have shown that the D2:D4 ratio is significantly smaller (and therefore similar to the ratio observed in men) in lesbians than in heterosexual women, which is in perfect agreement with the theory that assigns a role for prenatal hormones in the development of homosexuality (McFadden & Shubel, 2002; Rahman & Wilson, 2003c; Kraemer et al., 2006). This difference was recently confirmed by a meta-analysis of multiple studies involving thousands of subjects (Grimbos et al., 2010). It was also shown that only lesbians who identify as masculine (known as "butch") have this decreased D2:D4 ratio (Brown et al., 2002a). Another study also confirmed these results independently, showing that among monozygotic twins (true twins), where one is homosexual and the other not, the lesbian sister had a smaller (masculine) D2:D4 ratio compared with the heterosexual sister (Hall & Love, 2003). This work also shows that these variations of the D2:D4 ratio are independent of genes, since the study is of twins that have an identical genetic heritage. A more recent study based on a larger number of subjects, however, indicates a genetic contribution in conjunction with a contribution of the prenatal environment in the determination of the D2:D4 ratio (Gobrogge et al., 2008). These studies therefore imply that if testosterone is a key factor that determines this ratio, twins may be exposed to different concentrations of testosterone, which so far has not been experimentally tested. However, it is also possible that the twins could be exposed to the same concentration of steroids but be differentially sensitive (e.g., differences in the density of androgen receptors in the intracellular metabolism of the hormone, etc.; see Chapter 3). To my knowledge, only one study has not replicated the relationship between the D2:D4 ratio and sexual orientation in women (Lippa, 2003a).

Four similar studies were conducted among men, in whom it could be expected that homosexuality is associated with a more feminine (higher) D2:D4 ratio, with conflicting results (only one of the four studies conducted among men jibes with the predictions of the prenatal hormonal theory).

Differences in the Length of Various Long Bones

The growth of the bones of the hand seems to be under the control of embryonic steroid hormones, which would explain the sex difference of the D2:D4 ratio and the modification of this ratio in homosexual women, which would be due to their exposure to an abnormally high concentration of androgens during fetal life. Pursuing this idea further, researchers looked at the lengths of various long bones in males and females and the changes in the relationships between these lengths in homosexual individuals (Martin & Nguyen, 2004). This study was conducted to test the hypothesis that these ratios could be a reflection of the embryonic hormonal environment (androgenic and/or estrogenic) and thus provide information on the potential hormonal causes of a reversal of sexual orientation.

It was shown that the length of the bones that become sexually dimorphic in infancy was significantly different between homosexual and heterosexual individuals, while the bones that become different between men and women after puberty are not modified according to sexual orientation. Thus, people who have a sexual preference for men (heterosexual women and homosexual men) have a smaller growth of the bones of the arms, legs, and hands than subjects who have a sexual preference for women (heterosexual men and homosexual women). These data support the idea that gay men have experienced a reduced exposure to sex steroids during development, and conversely that the homosexual women were exposed to higher concentrations of sex steroids than heterosexual women, or alternatively that the sensitivity to these hormones is different in relation to sexual orientation.

Before this major study based on over 500 subjects (Martin & Nguyen, 2004), other less systematic work had already identified in males differences in ratios of the lengths of various parts of the body associated with sexual orientation [see references in Martin & Nguyen (2004)]. It is therefore quite likely that the results of this study are reproducible.

Other studies have identified differences compatible with the existence of endocrine disruption during development in homosexuals, but they appear to be less reproducible at the present stage of knowledge. These studies should certainly be pursued.

PHYSIOLOGICAL DIFFERENCES

Oto-Acoustic Emissions

It was discovered in the late 1970s that the inner ear, in addition to its obvious function in hearing, also emits sounds in the form of barely audible clicks that can be recorded by placing a sensitive microphone in the canal of the ear. The subjects do not usually hear these sounds, which are called oto-acoustic emissions (OAE). They are produced either spontaneously or in response to external short noises (e.g., clicks; Figure 8.2). It is interesting, for the purposes of this book, that oto-acoustic emissions are different in men and women. Women produce more oto-acoustic emissions, with a greater amplitude, than men do in the same situation. This difference is already present during childhood. The functional significance of oto-acoustic emissions is unclear (they seem to be an indirect consequence of the functioning of the inner ear), but it is thought that the sex difference that affects this sound production is largely the result of the prenatal exposure to androgens in male embryos (McFadden, 2002; 2011).

This hypothesis is supported by studies of OAE in animals. These OAE are indeed found, *mutatis mutandis*, both in sheep and in monkeys, and they are

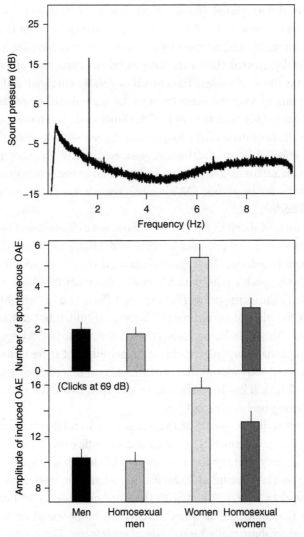

Figure 8.2 The oto-acoustic emissions (OAE) are sexually differentiated and significantly masculinized in homosexual females. The upper figure shows the distribution of frequencies and amplitudes of a spontaneous OAE recorded directly into the ear canal. The individual has a peak of emission at 1,700 Hz. Some individuals have such peaks at multiple frequencies. The lower figure represents the average number of spontaneous OAE and OAE amplitude evoked by clicks sounds measured in the right ear of hetero- or homosexual males and females (according to McFadden, 2002; 2008).

also sexually differentiated (female OAE are more frequent and of greater amplitude than in males). OAE were studied in hyenas because in this species, females are strongly masculinized by androgens during fetal life and immediately postnatally, so that their external genital structures are at first sight not different from those of males. The clitoris is greatly enlarged and, for a naïve observer, seems to have the same form as the male penis. Correspondingly, it was noted that in this case, the OAE of the females do not have a greater magnitude than those of males. This magnitude is even slightly lower. The OAE of hyenas are affected by prenatal androgens, because if pregnant mothers are treated with an antiandrogen (compound that blocks the action of androgens at their receptor), an amplitude OAE well above normal is observed in treated young (McFadden, 2008).

Furthermore, in sheep that show the classic sex difference in OAE (female > male), it was shown that prenatal treatment of female embryos with testosterone considerably reduced the magnitude of their OAE (McFadden et al., 2009). Finally, in both species (sheep and hyena), castration in adulthood does not affect the OAE, thus confirming that the sex difference affecting this characteristic reflects the physiological prenatal hormonal milieu but not activation by steroids in adulthood. In humans also, the sex difference in OAE seems to result mostly from prenatal organizing effects of steroids, but there is also some evidence for limited activational effects of steroids on this physiological response (McFadden, 2011). It has been shown, for example, that OAE are masculinized in women taking oral contraceptives.

Researchers at the University of Texas at Austin found that lesbians and bisexual women have oto-acoustic emissions and acoustic evoked potentials that are partially male: they emit significantly fewer OAE than heterosexual women, and these OAE have a lower amplitude (McFadden & Pasanen, 1998; 1999; McFadden, 2002). These data are consistent with the hormonal theory of homosexuality stating that female fetuses destined to become homosexual or bisexual have been exposed to abnormally high levels of androgens. These same researchers also demonstrated that women who had a twin brother and therefore had potentially been exposed to slightly higher levels of testosterone during embryonic life (testosterone produced by the twin would have diffused to the female embryo) had masculinized OAE, thus confirming sensitivity to androgens of the response in humans. However, the same researchers found no difference between the OAE of homo- and heterosexual males.

Evoked Acoustic Potentials and Alarm Response ("Startle Response")

The same group of researchers in Texas also showed that the evoked acoustic potentials (electrical responses induced in the brain by short auditory stimuli) are also different in men and women, and in (partly masculinized) homosexual or bisexual women compared with heterosexual women. By contrast, other characteristics of these evoked acoustic potentials were hypermasculinized in homosexual men when compared with values observed in heterosexual men (McFadden & Champlin, 2000). This study is again consistent with the idea that lesbians were exposed to abnormally high levels of androgens during fetal life but that, contrary to what one might intuit, gay men have been masculinized as much or even more than heterosexual men. Indeed, if we remain in the context of an interpretation based on differences in the concentrations of testosterone that embryos have been exposed to, we should conclude that if lesbians were exposed to concentrations higher than heterosexual women, they would have been masculinized and therefore present a male-typical sexual orientation (preference for women), which is consistent with the theory. In contrast, these data would suggest that gay men were exposed in utero to testosterone at above-normal levels. No definitive explanation for these paradoxical observations about gay men has been provided to date, but several potential mechanisms have been suggested (McFadden, 2011). Since it is a recurring paradox that I have noted before, it may be that we still have an imperfect understanding of some hormonal effects.

An independent study in London has also focused on the analysis of another physiological response known to be sexually differentiated—the particular fear response called the alarm or startle response. Following a loud noise, there is a blink of the eyes, but this response is partially inhibited if the loud noise is preceded by a lower noise. This inhibition by the preceding sound (prepulse inhibition) is usually less pronounced among women than among men. The group of Rahman and his colleagues recently showed that inhibition of the blink by a low alarm is stronger among lesbians than among heterosexual women (Rahman et al., 2003b). This response is masculinized in agreement with the prenatal hormonal theory of homosexuality. However, here again, the authors have not found this difference in inhibition between homosexual and heterosexual men.

Positive Feedback in Response to Estradiol

In rats and many other mammals, ovulation is induced in females by a gradual increase in plasma estradiol during the follicular phase of the cycle. When these concentrations reach a threshold, they induce a positive feedback resulting in a significant peak of release of luteinizing hormone (LH), which is responsible for ovulation, among other functions. The LH peak can be artificially induced in females by a single injection of a high dose of estrogen, but males are unable to produce such a peak of LH in response to estrogen. This neuroendocrine sex difference is organized during the embryonic and perinatal period by the same hormonal mechanisms that differentiate sexual behavior. The male embryos are masculinized and defeminized by early exposure to testosterone, whereas the female phenotype develops in the relative absence of hormones (Chapter 3). The injection of testosterone in female embryos of rats induces the loss of the LH peak in response to estradiol, but males castrated immediately after birth are able to produce such a peak.

Having suggested that human male homosexuality could be the result of inadequate masculinization during embryonic life, Dörner wondered whether the positive feedback of estrogen on LH secretion might be different in homosexual and heterosexual males (Dörner, 1969). In women, an estrogen injection at an appropriate time of the ovarian cycle induced a strong increase of circulating levels of LH, whereas this response was not observed in men. In keeping with his theory, Dörner showed that gay men react to an injection of estrogen by a significant increase in blood levels of LH. This increase is lower than that observed in women, but it is still significantly higher than among heterosexual men (Dörner, 1972; 1976; 1980).

These publications raised a huge controversy, in part because of the researcher's views concerning preventive treatments that he suggested should be established to prevent the emergence of gays, but also because the positive feedback of estrogen on LH that is quite evident in the rat is apparently not present in monkeys (Baum et al., 1985), a finding that raises the question of its existence in humans. Many researchers have thus doubted the reality of the effect identified by Dörner. In an attempt to resolve this controversy, American neuroendocrinologist Brian Gladue therefore decided to test the reproducibility of the effect. In a study published in *Science* in 1984, Gladue and colleagues clearly demonstrated the reproducibility of the effect identified by Dörner. After a single injection of Premarin, a compound with estrogenic action, women showed a major increase in LH 72 to 96 hours later (Gladue et al., 1984). This increase was not observed in men, but again an increase of intermediate magnitude was observed in men who reported having had a homosexual orientation during their life (see Figure 8.3).

This LH response to the injection of an estrogenic compound looks similar, but is not identical, to the positive feedback observed in the control of ovulation in rats [see for discussion Baum et al. (1985)]. It is important that there is a difference in this endocrine response in men according to their sexual orientation. However, based on available data, it is impossible to know whether this difference concerns a sexually differentiated neuroendocrine mechanism, which would suggest that homosexuals were exposed to "abnormal" endocrine conditions during their ontogeny. Alternatively, the differential response of LH to estrogens might just reflect a stable but unidentified difference in adult testicular

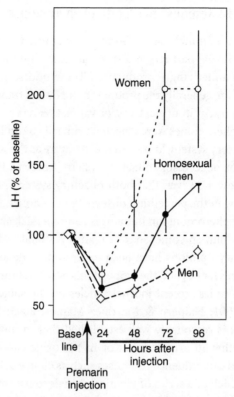

Figure 8.3 Changes in blood levels of luteinizing hormone (LH) in response to injection of a single dose of an estrogenic compound (Premarin) in heterosexual men and women and in homosexual men. The injection induced in women after 72–96 hours an increase in LH that was not present in men but was seen in an attenuated form in homosexuals (according to Gladue et al., 1984).

activity that could interfere with the positive and negative feedback on LH (Baum et al., 1985; Gladue, 1985).

Further studies should be conducted on this issue, but the fact remains that all this work indicates the existence of a (neuro)endocrine difference between homosexual and heterosexual men. We cannot conclude, at present, that this difference concerns a neuroendocrine mechanism, located most likely in the hypothalamus, that is known in rats to be differentiated (defeminized) during ontogenesis after exposure to testosterone rather than an aspect of testicular physiology associated in a less specific or even unknown manner to the differentiation of sexual behavior and brain. In either case, these data demonstrate the existence of a difference in the function of the hypothalamic-pituitary-testicular axis associated with homosexuality.

Brain Activation in Response to (Putative) Pheromones

In many species of mammals, some body odors emitted by males or females specifically attract sexual partners and stimulate (or inhibit in some situations) hormonal activity underlying reproduction. These odors, grouped under the term pheromones, are generally the product (more or less transformed) of sweat glands or may be present in urine, feces, or vaginal secretions. It was traditionally accepted that pheromones were detected primarily by an independent, auxiliary olfactory sensory system, known in the literature as the vomeronasal organ or organ of Jacobson or accessory olfactory system (Keverne, 1999). More recent studies tend to show, however, that both olfactory systems, the main and the auxiliary, play a role in the perception of sexual pheromones.

The existence of pheromones in humans is controversial, and many researchers believe that the human vomeronasal organ is vestigial and completely nonfunctional. Contrary opinions have been expressed. A detailed discussion of this controversy goes far beyond the scope of this book, but the interested reader may consult more or less recent journal articles on the subject (Foidart et al., 1994; Meredith, 2001; Halpern & Martinez-Marcos, 2003; Wysocki & Preti, 2004). However, it is reasonably well established that in humans, some compounds present either in armpit sweat or in the urine can be detected, consciously or not, and can influence responses such as choice of location (chairs in a waiting room; which of a series of identical urinals to use) and/or can modify the physiology and mood of subjects, even their sexual motivation. Experiments highlighting these effects are numerous and clearly not easy to replicate. They do not usually determine whether perception involves the main olfactory system or the vomeronasal system.

This problem is of little importance for what concerns us here, namely the possible difference of reaction to pheromones depending on heterosexuality or homosexuality. It was shown that the male rat brain is activated by the odor of bedding soiled by females, but no brain activation was observed in males exposed to bedding soiled by a male (Chapter 4). A perinatal treatment with a compound that blocks the aromatization of testosterone into estradiol irreversibly transforms a young rat into an adult male who is bisexual or homosexual and who will display behavior of sexual receptivity when placed with another male (Bakker et al., 1993a). In these subjects with a reversed sexual orientation, brain activity will correspondingly be stimulated by the smell of litter soiled by a male rat. Early hormonal treatment has therefore changed the brain activity in response to olfactory stimuli from an individual of the same sex (Bakker et al., 1996a).

In recent years, through advances in medical imaging techniques that can now detect which brain areas are activated during the presentation of a specific stimulus (among other things), researchers were able to identify a similar phenomenon in humans. Though this idea is disputed, two compounds derived from steroids are considered by some to be pheromones in humans: 4, 16-androstadien-3-one (AND) derived from testosterone in men, and the estrogenic compound estra-1, 3,5 (10),16-tetraene-3-ol (EST) in females. AND was identified in armpit sweat in humans, while EST is present in urine in women. The effects of these compounds appear to vary depending on the dose and the study protocol, but they have been shown to act on the autonomic nervous system and to alter mood and sexual arousal depending on context. Using two separate techniques of medical imaging, positron emission tomography (PET) and functional nuclear magnetic resonance (fMRI), a group of researchers from the Karolinska Institute in Stockholm have asked whether these compounds produced a differential activation of the brain in men and women and, if so, whether this activation was affected by the sexual orientation of the subjects. In a first step, differential brain activations in the two sexes have been identified (Savic et al., 2001). In males, exposure to EST (but not to AND) induced activation of the anterior hypothalamus, a brain area clearly involved in the control of male sexual behavior. Among women, a hypothalamic activation was detected after exposure to AND but not to EST (Figure 8.4).

More recently, researchers have analyzed the association of these differential brain activations with the sexual orientation of the subjects. They were able to show a profoundly altered activation in homosexual men. Specifically, the preoptic area and hypothalamus were significantly activated by the perception of AND (a male stimulus) in gay men as in heterosexual women, but not in heterosexual men. In contrast, exposure to EST, a female stimulus, activated hypothalamic areas in heterosexual men but not in heterosexual women or homosexual men (see Figure 8.4) (Savic et al., 2005; Berglund et al., 2006).

Similar results have been observed in parallel in homosexual women in whom hypothalamic areas are not, contrary to what is seen in heterosexual women, activated by the male odor AND. One does not see in lesbians an activation by the female olfactory stimulus, EST (Berglund et al., 2006). These results show that the brains of homosexual men and women are differentially activated by odors with sexual connotations compared to the brains of heterosexual subjects of the same gonadal sex. The interpretation of these results is complicated by the fact that the olfactory stimuli were used in the experiments at high concentrations (crystalline form of the steroids), presumably much higher than what could ever be encountered in the real world. It is therefore difficult to ascertain whether similar differential reactions would be observed with biologically relevant concentrations. Furthermore, the data do not indicate, whether the differential perception of these odors with a sexual significance is the cause or the consequence of the sexual orientation of the subjects tested. One can indeed imagine that the smells produced by an individual can activate brain areas involved in sexual motivation among homosexuals of the same sex and therefore encourage a homosexual attraction,

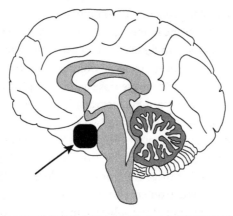

	Heterosexuals		Homosexuals	
	Men	Women	Men	Women
AND	−	+	+	−
EST	+	−	−	−

Figure 8.4 Exposure to potential pheromones differentially activates the hypothalamic area of males and females, and the response is modified based on their sexual orientation. The upper figure presents a schematic view of a sagittal section of human brain showing the region (arrow and black square) where metabolic activations were detected by medical imaging. The table indicates whether these hypothalamic activations are present (+) or absent (−) depending on the sex of the individual, his or her sexual orientation, and the compound used. AND = compound produced by men; EST = compound produced by women (according to Savic et al., 2005; Berglund et al., 2006).

although these odors would have no effect among heterosexuals. Conversely, it is also conceivable that being gay produces a sensitization to certain type of odors from individuals of the same sex and that this learning is reflected at the level of brain activity detected by medical imaging. By analogy with animal data, however, one might choose the first of these interpretations.

DIFFERENCES IN BRAIN STRUCTURE

As we have seen in the section on animal studies (Chapter 3), several limbic and hypothalamic nuclei involved in the control of sexual behavior are sexually differentiated. They are either larger in males than in females [sexually dimorphic nucleus (SDN) of preoptic area, bed nucleus of the stria terminalis (BNST)] or more developed in females than in males [antero-ventral nucleus of the anterior hypothalamus (AVPV), ventromedial nucleus of the hypothalamus (VMN)].

Researchers have questioned whether homologous nuclei, or at least nuclei located at the same places of the brain, were sexually differentiated in humans and whether the volume of these nuclei was modified according to the sexual orientation of the individuals. It is known that the volume of several of these nuclei (SDN, BNST, AVPV) is determined in rats by the action of sex hormones during the embryonic or immediately postnatal period and cannot be modified during adulthood. If that were the same in humans, the volume of these nuclei could then represent a reliable marker of the hormonal milieu in which an individual developed. If these nuclei were modified according to the sexual orientation of individuals, they would provide an additional argument concerning the validity of the hormonal hypothesis of sexual orientation.

The experimental material necessary to conduct such studies is very difficult to obtain. Structures that interest us here have a small volume and still cannot be identified by the in vivo imaging techniques currently available [magnetic resonance imaging (MRI) or positron emission tomography (PET)]. Only studies of postmortem tissue can provide useful information, and they have only been performed so far by a limited number of researchers with the few samples available in the human brain banks around the world. Some very interesting results have nevertheless been identified. They mainly concern the suprachiasmatic nucleus (SCN), the anterior commissure, and the sexually dimorphic nucleus of preoptic area (SDN-POA).

The Suprachiasmatic Nucleus

Morphometric analysis performed on a group of 18 heterosexual men who died of various causes and ten homosexual men who died of various diseases related to AIDS have shown that the SCN was significantly larger (1.7 times) in homosexuals than in heterosexuals (Swaab & Hofman, 1990). This nucleus in homosexuals also contained about two times more neurons than in heterosexuals. Thinking that the difference could be related to the indirect consequences of AIDS, these researchers also analyzed the SCN of six heterosexual men who died of AIDS and found that these subjects had a perfectly normal size SCN typical of heterosexuals.

This was the first study to demonstrate a neuroanatomical difference related to sexual orientation. As such, it deserves to be mentioned because it provided an important argument in favor of the idea that homosexuality is associated with specific biological changes. However, this neuroanatomical difference does not provide information about the mechanisms that lead to homosexuality. Although SCN, which is mainly related to the control of circadian rhythms, seems to be involved in the control of certain aspects of reproduction (Swaab & Hofman, 1990), there is no data suggesting a direct involvement in the control of sexual orientation (Kruijver et al., 1993). And since there is also no evidence that the volume of the SCN is sexually differentiated (greater or smaller in men than in women), the difference observed between homosexual and straight men does not provide any argument that might suggest a lack of masculinization of the brain.

The Anterior Commissure

The anterior commissure is the bundle of fibers that connects the two cerebral hemispheres in the anterior hypothalamus. A study of the brains of 90 subjects (heterosexual men and women and homosexual men) showed that this connection is significantly more developed in women than in men when measured in the mid-sagittal plane (Allen & Gorski, 1992). Moreover, the size of this anterior commissure is larger among homosexual men than among heterosexual men and even than in women (Figure 8.5). The anterior commissure is in fact 34% bigger in homosexual men than in heterosexual men and 18% larger than in women.

This neuroanatomical difference associated with genital sex, and in men also associated with sexual orientation, could at least partly explain some gender differences observed in various cognitive tasks (such as visual-spatial skills and verbal tasks) and sex differences of functional lateralization (male brains seem more strongly lateralized than female brains). Furthermore, gay men are quite similar to women for some of these criteria (see earlier parts of this chapter), and the large size of their anterior commissure is perfectly correlated with their

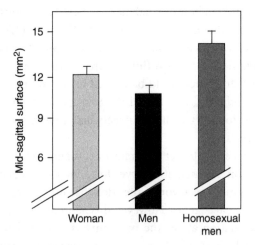

Figure 8.5 Size of the brain anterior commissure estimated from its surface in the mid-sagittal plane in men and women and in homosexual men (redrawn from Allen & Gorski, 1992).

cognitive abilities. However, some studies have failed to confirm these differences in cognitive abilities between heterosexual and homosexual men, so they must be treated with caution even though many aspects of experimental protocols, and in particular the selection of subjects, are likely to explain these failures of replication.

It is important to note here, once again, that the neuroanatomical difference in gay men affecting the size of the anterior commissure, a structure that has no direct link with sexuality, is an additional strong argument suggesting that homosexuality is not the result of a choice, but instead a complex phenotypic change that goes far beyond the field of sexuality and has in all likelihood biological bases beyond the control of the individuals.

The Corpus Callosum

In 1982, biologist Christine de Lacoste-Utamsing and her colleague Ralph Holloway published an article based on the postmortem study of human brains showing that another connection between the left and right cerebral hemispheres differs as a function of gender. The corpus callosum is by far the most important interhemispheric connection in humans (de Lacoste-Utamsing & Holloway, 1982). de Lacoste-Utamsing and Holloway showed that the shape of a part of the corpus callosum called the splenium was sexually differentiated, and was larger in women than in men. This work received enormous attention, and since the structure involved is large, it is possible now to view it by brain imaging in living subjects, thus making study much easier. Several studies have therefore addressed this question. Some could not reproduce the difference between sexes originally identified, while others have confirmed it. The existence of this difference remains controversial at present, but I shall not go into detail on the debate because it remains peripheral to the topic of this book.

However, a relationship between homosexuality and the shape of the corpus callosum has been identified recently and deserves our full attention. As I explained at the beginning of this chapter, male homosexuality is associated with a significant change in the manual lateralization: gay men are more often not right-handed (left-handed or ambidextrous) than heterosexuals. This unusual lateralization of the use of hands is itself normally correlated with increased size of the corpus callosum, especially its posterior part, called the isthmus. Researchers have therefore questioned whether the unusual lateralization in homosexual men (greater frequency of left-handers and ambidextrous) was associated with a difference in the size of the isthmus of the corpus callosum. To obtain results that are exclusively related to sexual orientation and are not simply a reflection of the manual lateralization, they compared the size of the isthmus by magnetic resonance imaging in 12 homosexuals and ten heterosexuals who were all strictly right-handed.

They observed that the isthmus of the corpus callosum was significantly greater among homosexuals, thus indicating that they have, like women, a less pronounced brain asymmetry than do heterosexual men. Right-handed homosexuals thus have a cerebral functional asymmetry less developed than in heterosexual men, and the motor lateralization is partially dissociated in these homosexuals from the cerebral lateralization. Moreover, during this same study, researchers were able to show that statistical analysis could correctly identify the sexual orientation of the subject in 21 cases out of 22 based not only on the size of the isthmus of the corpus callosum but also on the basis of different cognitive tests already mentioned in this chapter. These data demonstrate an association between a neuroanatomical structure and cognition, and join many other results that indicate the existence of anatomical differences between the brains of homosexual and heterosexual men that indirectly support the hypothesis of a biological basis to sexual orientation (Witelson et al., 2008). Remember also that being left-handed or right-handed is a characteristic that appears early in development (Hepper et al., 1991). This feature cannot be a personal choice. The fact that it is correlated with sexual orientation suggests that sexual orientation is determined early.

The Sexually Dimorphic Nucleus of the Preoptic Area

As explained earlier, homosexuality can be induced experimentally and irreversibly in the laboratory rat by altering the hormonal milieu of the embryo or the young pup just after birth (Bakker et al., 1993a; Bakker et al., 1996a). This change in sexual orientation in rats is associated with a decrease in the volume of a group of cells located at the base of the brain (SDN-POA), which is normally larger in males than in females and develops to a female size in male rats that have been made "gay" by the early hormone treatment (Houtsmuller et al., 1994).

One or more sexually dimorphic nuclei are also present in the preoptic area of the human brain. A preoptic nucleus significantly larger in men than in women was first identified by Dick Swaab and colleagues at the Netherlands Institute for Brain Research in Amsterdam in 1985 (Swaab & Fliers, 1985). This difference is not present at birth but gradually develops during the first 10–15 years of life and persists until an advanced age (> 80 years), although its amplitude tends to decrease with age (Swaab & Hofman, 1988). A comparative analysis of the size of this nucleus in the brains of homosexual men, however, identified no difference in volume compared to heterosexual men, although this study highlighted a difference in the volume of another nucleus as a function of sexual orientation of the subjects (see preceding section on the suprachiasmatic nucleus).

A few years later, researchers from the laboratory of Roger Gorski (who had identified the SDN-POA of rats) at the University of California, Los Angeles, analyzed again the human preoptic area and described four distinct cell condensations (nuclei) in this region. They called these nuclei the INAH 1 to 4 for the interstitial nuclei of the anterior hypothalamus. Two of these nuclei were found to be larger in men than in women (INAH 2 and 3) (Allen et al., 1989). It was shown a little later that the INAH 3 was significantly smaller in homosexual men than heterosexual men. Its average size was in fact similar to the size of INAH 3 observed among women (LeVay, 1991) (Figure 8.6).

Bill Byne's independent study based on different brains confirmed the reduced size of INAH 3 in male homosexuals compared to heterosexuals, though the magnitude of the difference observed in this replication was lower than in the first study of LeVay and thus not statistically significant (Byne et al., 2001). This study also showed greater cell density (more cells per unit volume) in the INAH 3 of homosexuals than in heterosexuals. The nucleus of homosexuals thus has a cellular composition identical to that of heterosexuals (same number of neurons), but the neurons are closer to each other on average, possibly because they have

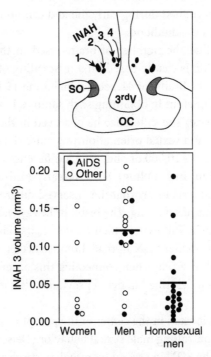

Figure 8.6 Schematic representation of the human hypothalamus illustrating the position of the four interstitial nuclei of the anterior hypothalamus (INAH) in relation to the 3rd ventricle (3rdV), the optic nerve chiasma (OC), and supraoptic nucleus (SO). The lower figure represents the values of the volume of INAH 3 measured in women, men, and gay men who died of AIDS or of another cause. The horizontal bars represent the average for each group of subjects (redrawn from LeVay, 1991).

formed fewer synapses during development. This observation and its interpretation, however, need to be confirmed.

Many critics have focused on the fact that many gay brains used in these studies came from individuals who had died of AIDS. It was therefore argued that the small size of the INAH 3 in these subjects arose from either AIDS or the intensive medical treatments to which these patients had been submitted. In the present state of knowledge, this critique is unfounded. Indeed, LeVay and Byne were perfectly aware of this problem and whenever possible included homosexuals in their samples who had died of a cause other than AIDS, as well as heterosexuals who died of AIDS. These data have not provided an argument to suggest that AIDS and its treatment can reduce the size of the SDN (see Figure 8.6). Thus, in the study of LeVay, the size of the SDN of heterosexuals who had died of AIDS was larger than the average size of that of homosexuals. In addition, the study of Byne and colleagues included nine heterosexual men who had died of AIDS and 22 who had died of other causes. A difference in volume of INAH 3 could not be detected between these two subgroups. It should also be recalled here that in rats, SDN size is determined during early life and can no longer be affected by any known treatment in adulthood.

It was also said that the number of brains used in these studies was too limited. This objection is clearly based on a misreading of the results. LeVay's study was based on the brains of 41 people, including 19 homosexuals, which given the difficulty inherent in obtaining such samples is a respectable or even remarkable sample size. The difference he observed in the volume of INAH 3 according to gender and sexual orientation was quite significant ($p < 0.00014$, or less than 2 chances in 10,000 of obtaining a difference of such an amplitude by random fluctuations in sampling). So it is clearly a misunderstanding of the meaning of statistical tests to say that the observed difference could simply be caused by fluctuations of sampling. The result of LeVay was by and large reproduced independently by Bill Byne, which reinforces its validity.

The presence of a smaller SDN in male homosexuals (IANH 3) acquires an especially important meaning when connecting this observation to the animal studies that have been described in detail previously. Remember the following:

1. The nucleus is located in the center of the preoptic area, which plays a key role in controlling male sexual behavior (Nelson, 2005).
2. The lesion of the SDN in several mammalian species induces a change in male sexual orientation from strictly heterosexual to either homosexual or bisexual (Paredes & Baum, 1995).
3. The larger size of SDN in males compared to females is determined exclusively by the action of sex steroids during embryonic and postnatal life (masculinization by testosterone and its estrogenic

metabolite, estradiol) (Jacobson et al., 1981; Arnold & Gorski, 1984; Rhees et al., 1990). Hormone treatments in adulthood have no effect on the size of the nucleus.

4. Perinatal treatment with an aromatase inhibitor that affects the sexual orientation of male rats (Bakker et al., 1993a; Bakker et al., 1993b) in parallel reduces the size of the SDN of the preoptic area (Houtsmuller et al., 1994).

5. In sheep, a smaller SDN of the preoptic area is associated with homosexual orientation of male sexual behavior (Roselli et al., 2004b), just as in humans. This nucleus also expresses less aromatase in homosexual sheep than in those who are sexually attracted to females. Recent experiments also indicate that, as in rats, the size of this nucleus in sheep is controlled by the action of testosterone during embryonic life (Roselli et al., 2007).

If these results of experiments on animals are transposed to the human SDN (INAH 3), the difference in the size of the nucleus observed in homosexuals is an argument to support the theory of an early hormonal origin of homosexuality. Homosexuality in the human male would be the result of the early exposure to low concentrations of testosterone. Small SDN in homosexuals would be the signature of this atypical embryonic hormonal environment and, given the role of the SDN in animals, could even be considered to be one cause—maybe *the* cause—of homosexuality.

However, there are a number of considerations that should temper the tendency to extrapolate too quickly from this finding.

1. The homology (strict identity) between the preoptic SDNs of rats, sheep, and humans is not established so far. The preoptic area has a complex architecture and in humans, in particular, four INAH were identified and only one is changed among homosexuals (INAH 3). The work of Swaab had identified another sexually dimorphic nucleus in the human anterior hypothalamus (Swaab & Fliers, 1985), which is likely to be equivalent to INAH 1 (LeVay, 1991), but INAH 1 was not shown to be larger in men than in women (Allen et al., 1989). Differences in sampling (different age of subjects in both studies) almost surely explain this discrepancy (Garcia-Falgueras & Swaab, 2008), but before we have a replication of these studies, this interpretation remains uncertain. It is therefore possible that the SDN identified in different animal species and humans are merely similar, not strictly homologous. Additional anatomical and neurochemical studies, admittedly complex but nevertheless possible, should help

answer this objection. But even if a strict neuroanatomical homology
were established between the human INAH 3 and the SDN in rats and
sheep, this would not demonstrate that all the characteristics of these
nuclei must be identical (see 2 and 3).

2. No studies are available (and probably will never be, for obvious
   logistical reasons) to demonstrate that the size of the human INAH 3 is
   determined exclusively by embryonic hormones. This is the case for the
   SDN in rats and also in sheep, but to date nothing ensures that the
   same conclusion is true in humans. The volume of most dimorphic
   nuclei in mammals is determined irreversibly by embryonic hormones
   acting during a defined critical period, but there are some exceptions in
   which the hormones can still change the size of a sexually dimorphic
   nucleus in adulthood [e.g., part of the amygdala (Cooke et al., 1999),
   the medial preoptic area in rat (Bloch & Gorski, 1988a; b)]. A recent
   study has also demonstrated that the size of INAH 3 is slightly reduced
   in human males castrated in adulthood for medical reasons (prostate
   cancer). Although the difference was not statistically significant, it
   remains possible that the volume of INAH 3 is at least partly
   determined by hormonal status in adults (Garcia-Falgueras & Swaab,
   2008). In addition, the study of Bill Byne suggests that the small size of
   the INAH 3 in gay people would not be accompanied by a decrease in
   the number of neurons but would rather result from their greater
   density (Byne et al., 2001). This seems different from what is known in
   rats, where the smaller SDN of females is due to enhanced neuronal
   death during development. Adult females have fewer neurons in SDN
   than males. It is therefore important to replicate this observation of Bill
   Byne in order to further assess how far the human–rat comparisons
   can be pursued in this area.

3. Although the human INAH 3 is located in roughly the same place as
   the SDN of rats, manipulation (e.g. lesion) has not been, nor will be
   for obvious ethical reasons, carried out to confirm that INAH 3
   indeed controls sexual orientation in humans.

4. The studies of LeVay and Byne cannot answer the question of
   whether the smaller INAH 3 in homosexuals is the cause or the
   consequence of their sexual orientation. When causal relations
   between brain and behavior are addressed, one is spontaneously led to
   think that the changes in structure or function of the brain determine
   changes in behavior rather than vice versa, but numerous studies have
   demonstrated that, contrary to beliefs that were widespread until very
   recently, the structure of the brain is plastic. For example, it was
   shown that if rats are raised in environments enriched with a more

complex spatial structure, the size of their hippocampus (a brain area heavily used for orientation in space) and the complexity of its neurons are increased as compared with control rats. Even in humans, it is established that the use of a specific area of the brain leads to its hypertrophy in a manner similar to the increase of the mass of a muscle that is highly used by an athlete.

One could thus imagine that the small size of the SDN in homosexuals is induced by an aspect of their behavior or lifestyle, rather than being the cause of their orientation. It has been observed that many homosexuals living in New York and California, from which came the subjects in LeVay's study, had sexual activity involving large numbers of relationships with many partners. One might therefore think that the smaller size of SDN could be the result of that intense and diversified sexual activity. This argument cannot be formally rejected, but all cases of behavior-induced plasticity in the nervous system that have been described both in animals and in humans never concern the hypothalamus and limbic system but instead are almost always related to the cerebral hemispheres. These brain areas seem to react to plastic life experiences of the subject, whereas the hypothalamus appears to be controlled by intrinsic physiological mechanisms based largely on hormonal changes. It is not excluded that in the future researchers will discover changes in the hypothalamus induced by experience, but in the current state of knowledge, data do not support this hypothesis.

In a minimalist interpretation, one can imagine that the small size of the homosexual INAH 3 represents a signature of the early hormonal environment in which these individuals have developed, but the size of the nucleus is not responsible for the sexual orientation of the individuals. In other words, the small size of the INAH 3 and the sexual orientation of the concerned individual would have both been induced by the presence of abnormal embryonic hormonal conditions (probably an overly low concentration of testosterone), but these two features would not be directly related in a causal manner.

Alternatively, if we consider that lesions of the preoptic area (including SDN) of rats or ferrets change their sexual orientation, it is also possible that there is actually a causal chain that, from a low level of embryonic testosterone, leads to the development of a small INAH 3 that is the cause of the homosexual orientation. To defend this hypothesis further, it should be previously determined by what mechanism a small SDN/INAH 3 can be the cause of a reversed sexual orientation.

Finally, we should note that even if we consider the latter interpretation of these data sympathetically, the fact remains that the size of INAH 3 and cellular changes that must necessarily accompany the changes in the volume of this nucleus cannot be the only cause of homosexuality. Indeed, although the average volume of INAH 3 in homosexuals is statistically smaller than in heterosexuals, there is some overlap between the volumes observed in both groups. In other words, the smallest of the INAH 3 observed in heterosexuals have a volume smaller than the largest nuclei observed in homosexuals. The size of this nucleus thus cannot be the sole cause of homosexuality. This feature may predispose to sexual orientation, but not produce it by itself.

PROBLEMS AND GENERAL INTERPRETATION

If we review all the studies presented in this section, it is clear that homosexuality in men and women is significantly associated with a range of physical, functional, and behavioral characteristics that are modified from what is normally seen in heterosexual individuals. These characteristics are not changed in all studies, however, and are not always observed in both sexes. The question arises, therefore, of why these correlations with independent markers of homosexuality are not stronger and more reproducible. Various factors probably contribute to obscuring the relationship.

1. Homosexuality is a complex phenomenon that may have multiple causes that are not the same in all individuals. Prenatal hormonal causes may concern only certain subjects, so the traits under study would be changed only in some homosexual individuals.

2. The classification of subjects as homosexual, heterosexual, or bisexual is often based on questionnaires or spontaneous statements. These answers may be biased for a variety of reasons, and the classification of individuals included in the studies could be partially wrong, which would dilute the relationship with the so-called "markers" of homosexuality.

3. The studies conducted so far have been unable to determine whether the hormonal difference supposed to lead to homosexuality is the embryonic concentration of circulating testosterone or the brain sensitivity to the action of this steroid. If the level of circulating testosterone is affected during a critical period of development of the sexual orientation, orientation will be affected, as well as all other androgen-dependent responses that are developing at the same time. If instead it is the sensitivity of the brain to testosterone that is changed but the circulating levels are normal, we can expect to find adult homosexual individuals in whom most physical or functional characteristics are identical to those of heterosexuals. Only neural or behavioral characteristics that depend on the same mechanism of sensitivity to androgens as sexual orientation will be affected. Both options are not exclusive. It is possible that for some homosexuals, there are correlations

with peripheral changes (if the circulating testosterone was affected) but that these correlations are not present among other subjects (for whom brain sensitivity to testosterone is changed).

4. The dose-response relationships that link the concentration of circulating testosterone during embryonic development with the mechanism controlling sexual orientation and its various correlates are not known and could be different. Studies of animal behavior and physiology have shown that among a group of responses controlled by hormones, some are affected by lower doses than others. If we imagine that human sexual orientation is more sensitive to small variations in testosterone levels than other hormonal responses described above (to which it is sometimes correlated), we can easily obtain homosexual individuals in whom the trait associated with homosexuality is affected (strong hormonal changes) and others for whom it is not (more subtle hormonal changes).

5. In the same way, the critical period during which sexual orientation and its various correlates are determined might be partially different, as is the case for various responses studied in animals. Hormonal events occurring at a specific stage of development can affect one response without affecting the others significantly. Since we know nothing of these critical periods, this possibility is difficult to assess. All the interpretations set out in items 3 to 5 of this list are derived directly from studies on animal models and could easily be tested on animals. In humans, obvious ethical reasons prohibit deliberate manipulations of embryonic hormones, and it is therefore much more difficult to obtain information on the mechanistic aspects of hormonal action during ontogeny.

6. Finally, any prenatal endocrine phenomenon that leads to homosexuality is obviously not completely deterministic but simply modulates the probability of occurrence of this orientation. It is possible and even likely that to determine sexual orientation in adulthood, it is necessary that various hormonal and biological changes accumulate in the same subject or that the predisposition to homosexuality induced by embryonic hormones is strengthened by not-yet-identified aspects of interaction with parents, teachers, or society in general. It is possible that a predisposition to homosexuality that would be controlled by prenatal biological factors can only be manifested in particular circumstances of the environment. These have not been identified. If these "social" influences exist, their importance is probably less than that of the embryonic hormonal factors, since they are so far much better identified.

9

Sexual Orientation in Clinical Cases

The previous chapter was devoted to the description of correlations identified between homosexuality and changes in sexually differentiated features. Although alternative interpretations are possible in some cases (and some cases only), the likely interpretation of these differences associated with homosexuality is that they result from hormonal changes that occurred during embryonic life that affected, in parallel, the sexual orientation and the development of characteristics normally differentiated between men and women. A real test of this causal interpretation would be to manipulate a group of randomly selected human embryos with steroid hormones and to analyze their sexual orientation 20 years later. This experience is of course morally proscribed. Nevertheless, there are various conditions described in detail in Chapter 6 that allow us to understand the impact on the sexual orientation of spontaneous hormonal changes in the embryonic environment in humans. Many studies have been devoted to this topic.

These variations are often called "invoked experiences," but they are in fact only pseudo-experiments because they do not affect individuals randomly, and one can never be sure that the hormonal variable that is studied is the only change compared to a group of control subjects and is therefore responsible for the observed effects on sexual orientation. This being said, given the ethical limitations associated with experimentation in this area, these pseudo-experiments probably represent the best possible source of information. The information that was collected using this approach will be considered here in detail.

EFFECTS OF PRENATAL STRESS

The first hormonal theory of homosexuality was developed by Günter Dörner, already referenced in this book several times. It was based on the results of animal studies conducted by Ingeborg and Byron Ward and their colleagues from Villanova University in Pennsylvania, showing that when pregnant rats are stressed (immobilization in a highly illuminated area), the sexual differentiation of young males from these mothers is significantly affected (Ward, 1972).

In rats, the distance between the genitals and the anus is smaller in females than in males. However, males born from these stressed pregnant rats have at birth a shorter distance between the base of the penis and anus than normal males. In adulthood, the males show atypical sexual behavior: they mount females less frequently and are even capable of presenting female-typical behaviors such as lordosis in response to sexual advances of other males (Ward & Ward, 1985). The volume of their sexually dimorphic nucleus of the preoptic area (SDN) is also lower than normal and thus closer to values typical of females (Anderson et al., 1985; Kerchner & Ward, 1992).

All these changes clearly reflect a partial lack of masculinization and defeminization. The analysis of the endocrine status of these embryos under stress has also revealed that their blood level of testosterone was reduced and, in addition, that the aromatase activity (conversion of testosterone into estradiol) was inhibited in their preoptic area (Weisz, 1983; Ward, 1984; Jimbo et al., 1998). These hormonal changes induced by stress and the associated increase in circulating levels of corticosterone were clearly responsible for their incomplete sexual differentiation (see Chapter 3).

Based on these results, and given that male homosexuality could be primarily considered as a lack of masculinization (like a heterosexual woman, a gay man is attracted to men), Dörner hypothesized that gay men should be born to mothers who were stressed during their pregnancy. He then performed retrospective studies by interview to research whether the mothers of homosexuals had experienced stressful events during their pregnancy with a higher frequency than mothers of heterosexual control subjects. The data collected showed that there was a significant peak in frequency of gay men among cohorts of boys born in Berlin between 1942 and 1946 (Dörner, 1980; Dörner et al., 1980; Dörner et al., 1983). This increase did not appear be linked to an increased reporting and detection of homosexuals linked to the appearance around 1970 of a more tolerant attitude toward homosexuality. Indeed, this peak is transient and is specific to pregnancies having taken place during World War II.

Mothers interviewed in this study lived in Berlin. It is thus easy to imagine that many of them had experienced extremely stressful events during pregnancy. A more detailed analysis of the questionnaires also indicated a relationship between highly stressful life events that mothers remembered and the likelihood that their boy born in this period be homosexual. Less than 10% of mothers of heterosexual boys had been exposed to stressful events, but more than 30% of mothers of homosexuals had been placed in such situations. Mothers of bisexual men occupied an intermediate position (Dörner et al., 1983). These data therefore suggest that stress experienced during pregnancy may increase the likelihood of homosexual orientation in males, probably due to an interference of corticosteroids (stress hormones) with the production or action of androgens or their estrogenic metabolites as described in the rat.

Animal studies by Ward and colleagues had not shown an effect of stress on sexual orientation but rather on the type of behavior (male or female) performed by the subjects. This was declared by some to contradict Dörner's results and conclusions. As I have explained before, these are two different dimensions of sexuality that should not be confounded. Since that time it was also shown that (1) the sexual orientation of rodents is controlled by hormonal embryonic mechanisms similar to those that control the expression of male-typical or female-typical behavior (see Chapter 4), and (2) that maternal stress affects the volume of the sexually dimorphic nucleus of the preoptic area and this nucleus seems to be involved in the control of male sexual orientation (Paredes et al., 1998). These data thus gave new importance to the observations of Dörner.

However, more recent studies have failed to reproduce the correlation between maternal stress and homosexual behavior observed by Dörner (Schmidt & Clement, 1990; Bailey et al., 1991) or they only produced equivocal data (Ellis et al., 1988). We can wonder, however, whether the importance of stress experienced by mothers during these more recent studies is really comparable to the stress that mothers were exposed to while living in Berlin during the Second World War during the intensive bombing of the city. In the present state of knowledge, the theory of prenatal stress as a factor to explain homosexuality does not seem firmly established in humans, even if it is applicable to the rat. These two species could obviously react differently to stressful situations from the endocrine and/or behavioral point of view. Additional studies would certainly be useful.

ANALYSIS OF WOMEN WITH ADRENAL HYPERPLASIA

Another source of information on the potential role of embryonic androgens in the control of sexual orientation may be found potentially in the study of girls with congenital hyperplasia of the adrenal glands (CAH) who have been exposed in utero to abnormally high levels of androgens (see Chapter 6). We have already seen that these girls display a masculinization of certain character traits during childhood, such as the type of toys used or drawings made freely (Berenbaum & Snyder, 1995; Berenbaum et al., 2000; Iijima et al., 2001). They also show a high level of physical activity, which is typical of boys.

There is an increase in CAH women of the probability of commitment or desire to engage in a homosexual relationship in comparison to a population of control females or to unaffected sisters of these androgenized women (Money et al., 1984; Dittmann et al., 1992; Zucker et al., 1996). Although there is an incidence of female homosexuality of 10–12% in a control population (Kinsey et al., 1953), or somewhat below 5% (Mosher et al., 2005), a study by John Money and his colleagues reported an incidence of homosexuality or bisexuality of 37% in CAH women (Figure 9.1). Recent studies have produced similar figures (Hines, 2006; Meyer-Bahlburg, 2009; Meyer-Bahlburg et al., 2008). A review by Meyer-Bahlburg and collaborators also presented a summary of 17 studies on the subject in which most studies showed an increased incidence of homosexuality or bisexuality in CAH girls.

The prenatal endocrine change corrected at birth is thus associated with a significant reduction of conventional heterosexual orientation. The explanatory interest of this medical condition is that postnatal treatment of the subjects

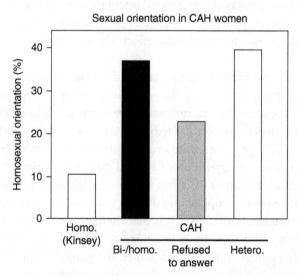

Figure 9.1 Effect of prenatal androgenization linked to the syndrome of congenital adrenal hyperplasia (CAH) on sexual orientation. One can observe in affected women a significant increase in the percentage of bisexual or homosexual orientation compared with control subjects and a large number of subjects refusing to answer questions relating to this topic (drawn from data in Money et al., 1984).

(as a girl) is expected to act in the opposite direction of the prenatal hormonal influence (masculinization). The masculinization of a behavioral trait (female homosexuality, or sexual attraction for women, a trait normally male) should thus in theory result from prenatal hormonal effects.

There are two possible alternative explanations, however, to this increased incidence of homosexual or bisexual orientation. First of all, the change of sexual orientation could be caused indirectly by the masculinization of the external genital structures. Although these were surgically corrected at birth, they still do not have an ideal structure in some women and therefore allow little or no penetrative heterosexual relationships. This could be one reason for engaging in homosexual rather than heterosexual relationships. It is also possible, theoretically, that the increase in nonheterosexual behavior and attraction in CAH women is induced indirectly by the reaction of the parents of the girl with masculinized genital structures. Even though these genital structures are surgically corrected at birth and adequate hormonal treatment is in place to block the secretion of androgens, the parents may not educate their daughter in the same way as an unaffected girl. However, one might reasonably assume that if parents have a modified reaction toward CAH girls, they should intentionally promote the feminine behavioral traits of these girls. Homosexual attraction in women is a trait normally found in men, and therefore one should expect that the action of parents would decrease this aspect of behavior. Since several studies have observed increased homosexual orientation in CAH girls, one would, in this interpretation, be lead to believe that parental efforts systematically produce an effect opposite to the intended effect. This would be paradoxical, to say the least.

Therefore, the most logical interpretation of the change of sexual orientation observed is that it was caused by the action of prenatal androgens. Of course, adrenal hyperplasia is a rare disease and cannot play a role in determining the sexual orientation of the majority of lesbians. Also note that the effect of prenatal androgens in CAH girls, even if it is very significant, has moderate amplitude. Only about 30% of the population of affected girls is not strictly heterosexual, and statistical calculation of the effect size of this difference (a measure of the difference with a control population taking into account the difference between means and the normal variation of this characteristic; see Chapter 5 for the definition of that term) demonstrates that it is five times smaller than the effect of the adrenal hyperplasia on children's games, for example (Hines, 2006). That said, the results nonetheless fit within the expected parameters.

The potential limits to the effects of embryonic androgens on sexual orientation might include the existence of limited periods of sensitivity to androgens that overlap only partially with the times during which these hormones are present in high concentrations in the blood (problem of time-response); the fact that children's games are more sensitive to androgens than sexual orientation (problem of dose-response); or finally that the part of the sexual orientation controlled by androgens is limited, and other prenatal or postnatal factors, including environmental or social and parental influences, are required. There is no way to discriminate between these interpretations at present.

TREATMENT OF PREGNANT MOTHERS WITH DES

Between 1939 and 1960, about two million pregnant women were treated with diethylstilbestrol (DES) in Europe and the United States to prevent an unwanted abortion. This treatment was not only ineffective but also damaging in that this substance, with its estrogenic activity, produces a slightly elevated risk of cervical cancer in girls exposed during their embryonic life. Studies suggest that, in addition, these girls have a greater likelihood of bisexuality or homosexuality (Ehrhardt et al., 1985; Meyer-Bahlburg et al., 1995; Swaab, 2007). Thus, the first of these studies showed that 24% of 30 women who were exposed to DES during their embryonic life were classified on the Kinsey scale (see Chapter 1) to scores of 2 to 6 (bisexuality or homosexuality), whereas none of 30 women used as controls in these studies (matched on as many variables as possible) were classified as bisexual or homosexual (Kinsey scores between 2 and 6) (Figure 9.2). Twelve of these girls had a sister not exposed to DES, and comparison of these

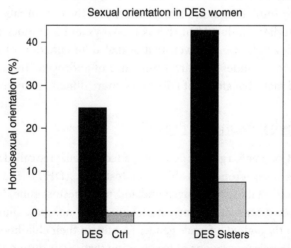

Figure 9.2 Effect of prenatal treatment with diethylstilbestrol (DES) on female sexual orientation. One can observe in treated women a significant increase in the percentage of individuals that are bisexual or homosexual as compared with control subjects. This increase is also reflected in the comparison of the subpopulation of women exposed to DES and their nonexposed sisters (drawn from data in Ehrhardt et al., 1985).

two populations also showed an increased incidence of bisexuality or homosexuality in subjects exposed to DES in utero (5/12 vs. 1/12).

A study by Meyer-Bahlburg and colleagues in 1995 similarly showed an increase of most measures of homosexual orientation (ideas associated with masturbation, dreams, attraction, relationships) in a population of DES women as compared with their controls, as well as in a subpopulation of sisters of whom only one of the two women had been exposed to DES before birth. In contrast, a more recent study suggests that girls exposed to DES before birth have a slightly lower probability (compared to control subjects) of having sex with a same-sex partner (Titus-Ernstoff et al., 2003). The origin of this discrepancy is unknown, but it could be related to the fact that this study considers only the actual sexual activity, whereas previous studies also analyzed other aspects of sexuality (fantasies, dreams) and used a graded scale (Kinsey scale in 7 points) rather than a dichotomous classification (presence/absence of a homosexual relationship).

If the effect of DES is real, which remains difficult to confirm given that this treatment has now been abandoned for a long time and the exposed subjects are becoming less and less available, this would indicate that estrogens as well as androgens (testosterone) are able to masculinize sexual orientation. This possibility is all the more likely given that in animals, testosterone exerts many of its effects on sexual differentiation after conversion into estradiol by aromatase in the brain (see Chapters 3 and 4). Furthermore, the potential effects of stress on human sexual differentiation described earlier in this chapter might be induced by inhibition of brain aromatase, as is the case in rats. It should be noted that studies conducted in rhesus monkeys and a number of data from clinical studies indicate, however, that sexual differentiation of the brain in humans would be under the direct influence of androgens (not aromatized), which would make the effects of DES much more difficult to interpret.

DEFICIENCY IN 5α-REDUCTASE

As we saw in Chapter 6, a genetic deficiency affects an enzyme called 5α-reductase that converts testosterone into dihydrotestosterone (DHT). The patients are exposed during fetal life to estrogen and androgen (testosterone) but not DHT. At birth, affected boys have poorly masculinized or nonmasculinized external genitalia, and they adopt a female gender identity in their childhood. Under the influence of massive secretions of testosterone that occur during puberty, their genitals are partially masculinized, and these children usually change their sexual identity in adulthood to live as men. This change of identity and gender role has even been observed in some individuals who had been married very young to a man as a girl and who remarried with a woman after puberty.

These studies have been criticized because children deficient in 5α-reductase are usually identified at birth. Terminology exists to name them in cultures where they live in substantial numbers (Dominican Republic and Papua), and one could therefore imagine that they are not really (fully) raised as girls, but rather as intersex individuals because their family knows that masculinization will occur at puberty (Rubin et al., 1981). Furthermore, it was also suggested that the sex change occurring at puberty was motivated by the privileges granted to men (especially in terms of independence, ability to undertake studies, etc.) in these relatively "macho" societies (Rubin et al., 1981).

Imperato-McGinley and her colleagues have shown that among 18 subjects from the Dominican Republic affected by that change who had completely female external genitalia at birth and had therefore been brought up in the firm belief that they were small girls, 17 have adopted a male sexual identity after puberty and became sexually attracted to women (Imperato-McGinley et al., 1991). The same authors have also reproduced these results in 5α-reductase-deficient subjects in Papua New Guinea, which is a much less indulgent society concerning the possibility of a change of gender identity and sexual orientation. Also in Papua, most affected children who had been raised unambiguously as girls changed their identity and sexual orientation after puberty (Imperato-McGinley et al., 1991).

Of course, many questions remain open regarding these studies. If we imagine that the change of identity and sexual orientation observed at puberty is the result of effects of androgens during fetal life (organizing effects) and puberty (activating effects) that are able to counteract the social experience and education of all young children almost completely, then we are led to believe that the action of testosterone on gender identity and sexual orientation is due to the hormone itself or its estrogenic metabolites and that conversion to DHT, the active metabolite at the peripheral level, is irrelevant for the behavioral responses. Also, the idea that these children are truly and fully raised as girls will always be impossible to prove. The fact remains that, as in the case of adrenal hyperplasia, if education has a role, it always leads to the opposite effect of what is desired by parents and thus also the opposite effect to be expected by those who say nurture trumps nature.

CLOACAL EXSTROPHY

Cloacal exstrophy is a rare, complex, genito-urinary malformation occurring during embryonic development that results in the birth of XY males who, in addition to various malformations of the pelvis, have no penis. This is not an endocrine disease, in that the testes are apparently normal both physically and functionally. In many cases, the XY individuals are assigned at birth a female sex both at the legal and social levels. They are also subjected to corrective surgery, including removal of the testes and vaginoplasty. Several recent studies have followed the psychosexual development of affected subjects, and one study observed that in a significant number of cases (sometimes up to 55%, 8/14), adult subjects chose to adopt a male identity and gender role (Reiner & Gearhart, 2004; Meyer-Bahlburg, 2005). A clear masculinization of games played by these XY children reared as girls was also present [preference for highly physical sports (football) or aggressive sports (karate)] (Schober et al., 2002; Reiner & Gearhart, 2004). In many cases, a typical male sexual orientation (attraction to women) was also observed.

These data again suggest that hormonal imprinting of the embryo by androgens could be responsible, at least in part, for the determinism of sexually differentiated characteristics such as gender identity and sexual orientation. This would result in a significant increase in the change of gender identity and sexual orientation later in life in subjects exposed in utero to androgens, despite the fact that they have subsequently been raised as girls. This change, however, does not concern all individuals. If this type of change is consistent with a role of prenatal androgens, it also indicates that androgens are probably not the only determinant and the postnatal environment is potentially also involved. I will come back to this idea.

OTHER ACCIDENTAL CHANGES IN THE EMBRYONIC HORMONAL MILIEU

The four conditions affecting sexual orientation described above contribute to the explanation of this feature because the assumed role of hormones goes against the supposed role of education. It is therefore possible to differentiate these two influences. There are also other endocrine changes that affect sexual orientation and put it into conflict with the genetic sex of the affected individuals, but these clinical cases are less interesting for the purpose of this work, because in these cases, the effect of education is consistent with the effect of the endocrine disease and therefore one cannot easily distinguish their respective roles.

Thus, males (XY) affected by complete androgen insensitivity are born, as detailed in Chapter 6, with completely female genitalia. They are then raised as girls and in general adopt a female gender identity and a female sexual orientation (they are sexually attracted by men). Detailed monitoring of a group of these patients indicated that they were very satisfied with their sexual identity and their sex life in general (Wisniewski et al., 2000). However, it is impossible in these cases to know whether the gender identity and sexual orientation as women are the result of the postnatal education or of the lack of action of testosterone during embryonic life.

Similarly, various chromosomal abnormalities that have been discussed previously (XXY or XYY boys and XO girls, see Chapter 6) provide little information for understanding the control mechanisms of sexual orientation because the missing or supernumerary chromosomes contain many genes whose absence or presence could directly or indirectly influence sexual orientation. It is thus impossible to link sexual orientation with any certainty to a specific genetic or hormonal factor.

IN CONCLUSION

I have in this chapter reviewed a number of medical conditions that are all related, at least in part, to sexual orientation at odds with the genetic sex of the affected subjects. In several of these conditions, a sexual orientation was finally adopted that was in opposition to the sex assigned at birth, but was consistent with the type of presumed hormonal exposure during intrauterine life (attraction to men given absence of androgens and to women given presence of androgens during embryogenesis). Most of the effects described here were reproduced in independent studies on populations of unrelated subjects, which adds to their credibility. It must be recognized that, occasionally, these effects could not be replicated in other research. This is not necessarily surprising given the complexity of these problems, including the selection of subjects and their controls and the difficulties associated with an accurate determination of gender identity and sexual orientation in subjects whose education and hormonal history were potentially disturbed.

Taken together, these data suggest that embryonic hormones could, in humans as in animals, play a significant role in determining sexual orientation. This conclusion is consistent with the results presented in the previous section indicating that homosexual orientation is often associated with a change in physical, functional, or behavioral traits supposed to differentiate themselves under the influence of prenatal sex steroids.

The most convincing medical cases suggesting a role of embryonic hormones on sexual orientation are those in which hormonal effects and education are supposed to pull in opposite directions, such as in congenital adrenal gland hypertrophy, prenatal DES exposure, 5α-reductase deficiency, and cloacal exstrophy. As in any clinical study, it is impossible to be completely sure that the sex in which subjects were educated was entirely consistent with what was desired. It would be surprising that in all cases, parents have unintentionally encouraged the development of a sexual attraction and sexual identity that would be contrary to their intentions (XX girls with adrenal hyperplasia raised as girls who become attracted to girls, XY boys with 5α-reductase deficiency or cloacal exstrophy raised as girls but adopting male gender identity and male sexual orientation in adulthood). The data therefore suggest a contribution of the hormonal embryonic milieu in agreement with what has been described in rodents.

However, it should also be noted that the medical problems discussed in this chapter are not associated with a reversal of sexual orientation in all subjects, except for androgen insensitivity syndrome (but in this case it is impossible to separate the role of embryonic hormones from the role of education). In all studies of medical conditions where hormonal effects and education are supposed to act in opposite directions, only a fraction of individuals (often 20–40%) show a reversal of sexual orientation in agreement with the hormonal influence. One should thus imagine that the prenatal hormonal environment only predisposes to sexual orientations (and identities) but does not fully determine them. I discuss this issue after considering the possible genetic influences.

10

A Genetic or Immunological Mechanism Underlying Homosexuality?

If one accepts that homosexual orientation develops in whole or in part following an abnormal exposure to sex steroids during embryonic life, the question arises as to the origin of these anomalies. Three hypotheses have been advanced: (1) lowered circulating levels of testosterone in the embryo could follow an external event, such as an intense and chronic stress suffered by the pregnant mother, which would prevent the complete masculinization of a male embryo and thus induce homosexuality at adulthood, (2) random variations of hormone concentrations could take place in which the extremes would be exposed to concentrations sufficiently low (in men) or high (in women) as to induce a disturbed phenotype, (3) genetic differences could induce abnormal circulating levels of hormones, disruption of the brain's response to these hormones, or a direct effect on sexual orientation independently of any hormonal changes.

The first of these possibilities (prenatal stress) was considered in the previous chapter, so I shall not return to it here. "Random" fluctuations of androgen concentrations to which male or female embryos are exposed are also possible (hypothesis 2). No biological parameter is actually adjusted to a specific value and, on the contrary, they fluctuate around a mean value. One can therefore imagine that, although male embryos are exposed to average concentrations of testosterone that are greater than those found in female embryos, there is an overlap between the values observed in the two sexes. In parallel, there may be a minimum concentration of testosterone to establish a male typical sexual orientation, i.e., a sexual attraction toward women (Figure 10.1). Under these assumptions, it is obvious that individuals exposed to testosterone levels in the intermediate zone of recovery of male and female concentrations could logically adopt a homosexual orientation.

Even if we could draw blood to measure the concentrations of circulating testosterone in a human embryo without a risk of abortion, we would still need a clear idea of the critical moment when the differentiation of sexual orientation takes place to predict when assays of testosterone concentrations in embryos should be performed to predict their orientation, and this information is not available. It is therefore extremely difficult to evaluate this theory based on spontaneous fluctuations in concentrations of embryonic testosterone and to determine to what extent it can explain the observed cases of homosexuality.

Anyway, a hormonal explanation could never be final because it always leads to the next question, which is to identify the cause of unusual hormonal condition ("random" fluctuations within the physiological range considered in hypothesis 2 or genetic change in hypothesis 3). Intense research efforts have therefore been undertaken to attempt to identify individual genetic differences (mutations or specific genes inherited from parents) that influence sexual orientation in humans either directly or by the hormonal mechanisms described previously.

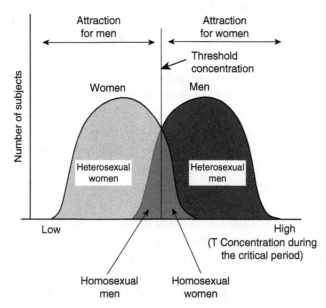

Figure 10.1 Model showing how the fluctuations around the average concentration of testosterone during embryonic life could lead to a homosexual orientation in a fraction of the population.

Given the complexity of the phenomenon studied, it is extremely likely that sexual orientation is not determined in a strict causal manner by a single gene. If this were the case, it is very likely that this gene would have been discovered by now.

It should be noted that some genes have a marked influence on all aspects of sexuality. Thus, certain recessive mutations in the gene controlling the synthesis of the androgen receptor lead to a complete lack of masculinization of the genetically male (XY) subjects who are affected (see Chapter 6). These individuals have female-typical external genitals, sexual identity, and sexual orientation. This orientation is homosexual if it is defined in relation to genetic sex (male), but it is in agreement with the physical and social sex and with the sex of education. This condition of androgen insensitivity illustrates the importance of certain genes in determining sex, but it is not a model of homosexuality in the conventional sense in which sexual orientation is in opposition to physical and sexual identity (and often education).

One can easily imagine the existence of more subtle genetic mechanisms (control of predispositions) depending on the interaction of several genes that may nevertheless play an important role in determining sexual orientation as such. Many studies indeed support the existence of such mechanisms.

THE CONCORDANCE OF SEXUAL ORIENTATION IN MONOZYGOTIC AND DIZYGOTIC TWINS

A genetic contribution to homosexuality was initially postulated on the basis that homosexuality tends to occur more frequently in some families than in others. Gay men on average have more gay brothers than heterosexual men. So in a given population, if a son is homosexual, between 20 and 25% of his brothers will also be homosexual, whereas if a son is heterosexual, the probability that his brothers are gay is only 4 to 6% (Diamond, 1993; Rahman & Wilson, 2003a). In parallel, lesbian girls have a higher probability (about 10% more) of having a sister that is also homosexual than do heterosexual girls. This correlation could of course result from psychosocial factors independent of genetics, but studies of twins allow us to reject this interpretation.

Many studies have actually compared the concordance of sexual orientation in matched pairs of twins. They all show that there is a much better concordance of orientation in true monozygotic twins than in dizygotic twins (fraternal twins born from different ova and sperm) (Figure 10.2).

The first study on this subject reported a rate of 100% concordance among identical twins but only 10% among fraternal twins. In other words, all monozygotic gay twins had a gay twin, but that was the case for only 10% of heterosexual twins. The selection of subjects in this study was probably suspect, but several

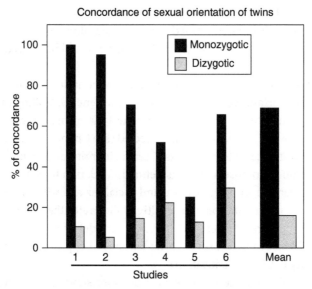

Figure 10.2 Percentage of concordance of homosexual orientation among true twins (monozygotic) or false (dizygotic) twins observed in six independent studies involving a total of 270 pairs of true and 271 pairs of false fraternal twins and average of the results. Note that a concordance of 100% does not indicate the presence of 100% of homosexuals in the population, but only that if in a twin pair one of the subjects was homosexual, the other was as well (according to data in Diamond, 1993).

more recent studies using more sophisticated methods of selection have resulted in a qualitatively similar conclusion showing a greater concordance of sexual orientation between true than in fraternal twins. Taken together, these studies indicate that 50–60% of the variance in sexual orientation in men is genetic in the socio-cultural conditions typical of Western societies (LeVay & Hamer, 1994; Rahman & Wilson, 2003a; Swaab, 2007). These studies may still be influenced by bias in the recruitment of subjects. Two recent very strict studies based on very large populations of Australian and U.S. twins show a concordance between monozyotic twins that is substantially lower, equal to about 30%. A separate analysis of Australian data also shows a concordance of 26% for men but 58% for women (see Rahman & Wilson, 2003a for more detail).

Whatever the precise value hiding behind these estimates, it is clear that all studies show a better concordance in real than in fraternal twins. This difference should be genetic. Identical twins in fact developed from the splitting of a single fertilized egg and therefore share (in first approximation) exactly the same genetic material, whereas dizygotic twins are not more similar genetically than siblings born at different times. This genetic identity is likely to cause the better concordance of sexual orientation. The only alternative explanation would be to assume that the two types of twins are raised in a different way (that is partially the case) and that these educational differences induce a better concordance in sexual orientation. Given the lack of data demonstrating a role of education on sexual orientation (Green, 1978), this interpretation seems unlikely at present. Absolute demonstration of the genetic interpretation of these data could be obtained by comparing two types of twins separated at birth, but due to the extreme rarity of this combination of already minority events (frequency of twins, homosexuality, separation at birth), this study will probably always remain impossible.

MATERNAL TRANSMISSION AND THE Xq28 REGION OF THE X CHROMOSOME

Studies of the potential genetic transmission of homosexuality through analysis of genealogical trees show that sexual orientation in men tends to be transmitted through the matriarchal line. In other words, a homosexual man has a higher probability of having gay men among his ancestors on the maternal side, but not on the paternal side. This type of inheritance may, of course, be explained in a simple way if one or more genes contributing to the emergence of homosexuality are located on the X chromosome (the only one inherited in a systematically different way from the father and mother). This maternal transmission was observed in three independent studies, but was not found in a fourth one.

The situation for women's sexual orientation seems more complex. Studies have identified an increased rate of nonheterosexuality (the term used to group homosexual and bisexual women) in girls, nieces, and cousins of the paternal lineage of lesbians. Such a transmission could also be consistent with a link to X chromosome, but it could come from the father as well as the mother. Other interpretations are also possible, and the interpretation of these data remains difficult (Rahman & Wilson, 2003a).

Molecular studies in gay men have subsequently attempted to identify the region of the X chromosome that might contain the gene(s) potentially linked to male homosexuality. On the basis of the genealogical tree of 114 families with gay sons, Hamer and colleagues confirmed the higher incidence of homosexuals in the maternal line (Hamer et al., 1993). In 40 families selected on the basis of containing two homosexual brothers and no indication of nonmaternal inheritance, they showed a correlation between homosexual orientation and the transmission of polymorphic markers located on chromosome X in more than half of the subjects tested. A detailed statistical analysis of these associations has finally shown a linkage with markers located in the subtelomeric region of the long arm of the sex chromosome, a region called Xq28. This association with the region Xq28 was found in two subsequent studies (Hu et al., 1995; Sanders & Dawood, 2003) but not in a fourth one (Rice et al., 1999). It should be noted

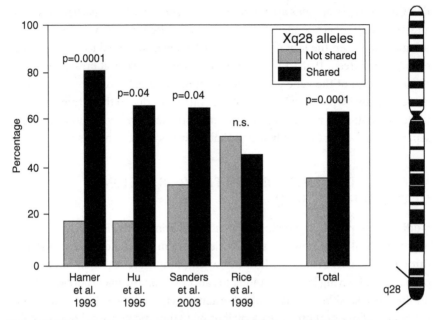

Figure 10.3 Four independent studies indicate a link between the transmission of male homosexuality and genetic markers located in the Xq28 region of chromosome X. The diagram on the right shows the location at the subtelomeric end of this set of genes on chromosome X (redrawn from Bocklandt & Vilain, 2007).

that this last study confirmed the link with maternal inheritance but had a lower statistical power and was therefore less likely to identify a significant link with Xq28 (Bocklandt & Vilain, 2007).

A comprehensive analysis of all available data, including negative results, however, indicates that approximately 64% of gay brothers have common alleles in the Xq28 region of chromosome X (Figure 10.3) (Bocklandt & Vilain, 2007). This association is significantly associated with a probability of less than 0.0001, which means there is less of a chance in ten thousand that the association appeared by chance in the data and does not reflect a real connection. That being said, it should be made immediately clear that this chromosomal region remains quite broad and could potentially contain many genes. We are still far from the identification of the responsible genes.

RESEARCH, SO FAR UNSUCCESSFUL, OF CANDIDATE GENES

To date, attempts to identify in the Xq28 region one or more genes that may contribute to the determinism of sexual orientation have all been unsuccessful (Bocklandt & Vilain, 2007; Ngun et al., 2011). Other approaches have been used to try unravel the genetic mechanisms potentially involved. A recent study has particularly been interested in the phenomenon of gene inactivation in the X chromosome. The male cells indeed contain a single copy of the X chromosome, while female cells contain two. So women (females) should theoretically produce a double amount of proteins whose genes are located on the X chromosome as compared to what is seen in men (male). To counteract this, each cell of a female embryo inactivates randomly one of the two X chromosomes. This inactivation is random in most cells, and it remains present in all cells that derive from a given cell in the adult tissues: all derived cells have one or the other X chromosome inactivated. Comparing this inactivation in mothers of homosexual or heterosexual sons, Bockland and collaborators have recently shown that inactivation showing an extreme asymmetry was present more frequently in the first group (13 of 97 = 13% in mothers of homosexuals) than in the second (4 of 103 = 4% in mothers of heterosexuals) and even more frequently in mothers of two or more gay boys (10/44 = 23%) (Bocklandt et al., 2006).

It is not known whether this unusual pattern of X chromosome inactivation is partly responsible for the homosexual orientation of the sons or is a consequence of an unidentified mechanism that directs this orientation. One possible explanation would be that one or more genetic factors that influence sexual orientation could also alter the survival of cells in the mother (white blood cells or stem cells), leading to a selection of cells that inactivate the one or the other allele. The fact remains that these data indicate that a mechanism that affects male sexual orientation is visible in the blood of the mothers. The unusual inactivation of the X chromosome among mothers of homosexuals also reinforces the idea that this chromosome influences sexual orientation.

The influence of the X chromosome is only partial and it is therefore likely that other genes located on nonsex chromosomes (autosomes) are also involved. A gene-linking study taking into account the entire genome was undertaken recently through advances in techniques of molecular biology (Mustanski et al., 2005). Unlike the studies focused on the X chromosome that only considered subjects with proven maternal transmission, this study did not use any criterion for exclusion of individuals. By mathematical techniques too complex to explain here, the study allowed for the identification of the maternal and paternal contribution to the transmission of homosexuality by the measure of a score called Lod (logarithm of odds). The largest parental genetic contributions to sexual orientation have been identified on chromosome 7 (position 7q36, maternal and paternal inheritance roughly equal) and chromosome 8 (position 8p12, again equal inheritance from both parents). An exclusively maternal effect was also identified on chromosome 10 (10q26). A similar study on a larger scale (more than 1,000 gay and heterosexual controls) is under way to confirm these results (see Bocklandt & Vilain, 2007; Ngun et al., 2011 for details).

The existence of a site of exclusively maternal heritability on chromosome 10 could lead to reinterpreting the results for the transmission of homosexuality through the maternal line. These results were interpreted as reflecting a transmission supported by the X chromosome, which is always inherited by a boy from his mother. It is also possible, however, that the transmission from mother to male child occurs by an autosome (chromosome 10 here) that would be altered by a change that does not affect the sequence of DNA, only its level of expression (called an epigenetic change). This involves changes (acetylation or methylation) of DNA and of proteins (histones) that surround it and results in the repression of the expression of certain genes. The repression is not necessarily identical on both chromosomes of a pair, which could explain these cases of exclusive maternal transmission through autosomes.

In an interesting way, this may also explain why there is not a complete concordance between orientation of monozygotic (true) twins. Although these true twins have in common all of their DNA, there might be differences in DNA methylation leading to differences in gene expression during critical periods of development (Fraga et al., 2005). The differences between monozygotic twins that are commonly attributed to specific effects of the environment could in fact be the result of a different epigenetic influence. This hypothesis opens up a new extremely large field of investigations.

THE OLDER BROTHERS EFFECT

The variable that has been linked in the most solid manner to male homosexuality is undoubtedly the number of older brothers born to the same mother. Although the mechanism by which this occurs has not been formally identified to date, it is likely that it involves at least in part a genetic contribution, and I therefore consider it in this chapter.

For over 20 years, Ray Blanchard and his colleagues at the University of Toronto and a few researchers working independently have shown that in humans, there is a highly reproducible correlation between the number of older brothers that a given subject (in this context, called the proband) has and the probability that he is homosexual. This effect has been called the "older brothers effect." An analysis of 14 independent studies representing more than 10,000 subjects found that for each additional older brother an experimental subject has, his probability of being gay increases by 33%. This does not of course mean that 33% of boys who have a brother born before them are gay, but that the likelihood of developing this orientation is 33% higher than in the general population. If we consider that the base percentage is 10%, the second son of a sibling will have a 13.3% probability of being homosexual (10 + 33%), the third 17.6% (13.3 + 33%), the fourth 23.4% (17.6 + 33%), etc. (Figure 10.4). The probability

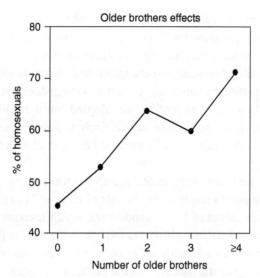

Figure 10.4 Relationship between the number of older brothers born to the same mother and the percentage of gay men in a population of 302 gay men and 302 heterosexual matched subjects used as controls. Because the homosexual and heterosexual subjects were matched for this study, there was 50% of homosexuals in the population studied, which is of course much higher than what is found in a normal population (redrawn from Blanchard & Bogaert, 1996).

that a fourth boy in a family is gay is thus about twice higher than for the first-born boy (Blanchard, 1997; Blanchard, 2004). Such a correlation could have many causes and interpretations. But given the robustness of the phenomenon and because it has been known for many years, it was possible by statistical analysis to exclude most of these alternative interpretations, and the authors of these studies now focus on an immune theory (Bogaert & Skorska, 2011), which I discuss below. Let us first consider all the most likely factors that have been considered but do not appear to explain this correlation.

It has been shown that the effect of older brothers is not observed for younger brothers (no increase in homosexuality, according to the number of brothers born after the proband) nor for sisters whether they are born before or after the proband. The effect does not depend on the number of brothers that were raised at the same time as the proband (a social effect that would be derived from an infancy spent with a lot of other boys) but only on the number of brothers previously born from the same mother (Bogaert, 2006). This effect is not found in girls. There is no increase in female homosexuality associated with the number of brothers or sisters born before (or after) the subject. All these data suggest a specific link with the sex of the children and that the sequence of births rather than the number of boys in a family is the relevant factor. This tends to show that the cause is not an educational factor but rather a biological factor associ-ated with multiple pregnancies. This notion is further strengthened by more recent analyses showing that the effect of older brothers (born before) is still observed if the subjects considered are raised in different families (because of divorce and reconstituted families), but that this effect does not occur for half-brothers (born to a different mother) or adopted brothers (Blanchard et al., 2006). These data therefore exclude, as effectively as possible in a psychological study in humans, the influence of postnatal educational effects of numerous siblings.

Furthermore, we know that parental age affects some characteristics of chil-dren, the best-known example being the rate of trisomy 21 (a genetic disorder that is one of two causes of Down syndrome), which increases with parental age. Since boys who have many brothers were born to mothers (and fathers) on average older than subjects with fewer older brothers, one would also have thought that the age of the parents was the explanatory factor. However, given the large samples (more than 10,000 subjects available), detailed statistical anal-ysis (by multiple correlations and partial regressions) could be used to reject this idea.

Having rejected over the years all the alternative hypotheses that could explain this effect, the only remaining explanation at present is based on a type of immune response of the pregnant mother. This interpretation considers that the mother who carries male embryos develops a progressive immune response over successive pregnancies against these embryos, which are considered a for-eign body that secretes foreign proteins in greater quantities than female embryos (Blanchard & Bogaert, 1996; Blanchard & Klassen, 1997). This is the hypothesis of progressive maternal immunization. The accumulation of antibodies is simi-lar to that seen if a Rhesus-negative mother sequentially carries in her womb several Rhesus-positive embryos. The first embryo is almost unaffected, but the following ones are quite severely attacked by the maternal antibodies and must often be prematurely removed from the uterus by Caesarean section or some-times have to undergo an complete change of blood at birth to prevent damage caused by maternal antibodies. The immune hypothesis to explain the effect of older brothers assumes that mothers who had boys previously produce antibod-ies against unidentified male proteins and that these antibodies affect the devel-opment of certain aspects of the brain that are involved in determining sexual orientation.

Consistent with this hypothesis, it was shown that the birth weight of boys with older brothers is significantly lower than the weight of matched boys with the same number of older sisters (Blanchard & Klassen, 1997; Blanchard, 2001). Moreover, within this population of subjects with older brothers, gay men had a lower body weight at birth than heterosexual men (about 6 ounces of difference, which is low but significant in the sample). These differences may be explained by the effects of hypothetical antibodies produced by the mother against the antigens typical of the male.

To mediate such an immune effect on the development of sexual orientation, a protein should theoretically fulfill a number of criteria (Bogaert & Skorska, 2011). Namely: (1) it should be expressed more or less specifically in the brain, since sexual orientation is obviously controlled by the brain and homosexuality is not associated with any major change in body structure or function, (2) it should be expressed at the surface of brain cells in order to be accessible to maternal antibodies, (3) it should be a protein specific to males, (4) fetal material containing this protein should enter the maternal circulation and should induce the formation of antibodies in the mother and (5) the concentration of these antibodies in the maternal circulation should increase with the number of male embryos that the mother has been exposed to. A small number of proteins have been identified that fulfill most of but not all these criteria. However, there is as of this date no formal proof that these proteins actually play a role in the control of sexual orientation and in particular in the increased incidence of homosexuality associated with the older brother effect. It is therefore premature to discuss these proeins here, but the interested reader can conveniently find a full discussion of this topic in a recent review (Bogaert & Skorska, 2011).

In summary, the mechanism underlying the effect of older brothers, and more specifically its immune aspects, remains unknown to date. It is possible to imagine an effect of the antibodies (which are known to penetrate the embryo) on the expression of genes and their interaction with the environment that are indispensable for the construction of an individual. However, there is no evidence of interaction with a genetic system, and the possible immune effects could result only from interactions with membrane proteins. Nevertheless, the effect of older brothers is without any doubt an argument of great weight supporting the idea that sexual orientation is significantly determined before birth.

EVOLUTIONARY SIGNIFICANCE OF HOMOSEXUALITY

Before closing the chapter, it is necessary to answer an objection frequently made about genetic theories of homosexuality. According to this objection, homosexuals do not reproduce, so if this orientation is controlled by one (or more) gene(s), this (these) gene(s) should disappear over the generations.

But it is wrong to say that homosexuals do not reproduce. It is important to recognize that some homosexuals change their apparent orientation during their life for various reasons often linked to social pressures (they hide their homosexuality until later in their life). During their apparent "heterosexual" phase, they may get married and eventually have children.

However, it remains clear, as proven by quantitative studies, that homosexuals reproduce less than heterosexuals. How is this lower reproductive success compatible with the maintenance of one or more genes controlling homosexuality? Several possible answers have been made to this apparent contradiction (Rahman & Wilson, 2003a; LeVay & Valente, 2006).

It is just possible that the gene or genes controlling homosexuality confers a reproductive advantage yet unknown, which would offset the negative effect on reproductive success of homosexuality as such. It is known that some genes have negative effects when they are present in the homozygous state (that is, on both chromosomes of a pair) but they confer a benefit on survival and thus reproduction when present on a single chromosome of the pair (heterozygous). The best-known example of this is sickle cell anemia, which causes a serious disease of the blood in the homozygous state but is associated with a resistance to malaria in the heterozygous state. Heterozygous individuals, because of the rules of genetics, are significantly more frequent than homozygous individuals, so that the gene for sickle cell anemia persists in the population, especially in malaria-infested areas where the advantage for survival is important. A gene favoring homosexuality could similarly be associated with an unidentified reproductive advantage in the heterozygous state (where homosexuality would not be apparent) but a clear decrease of the breeding success in the homozygous state.

It is also important to note that male homosexuality can be interpreted as an extreme attraction for males. If we imagine that the gene(s) controlling this trait of character has (have) a similar effect in women, the deleterious effect on male reproduction could be offset by an increased reproduction of women carrying the gene. Being more attracted to men, they would have a more intense sexual activity, resulting in a larger number of offspring. A fairly recent study showed that relatives (mothers, grandmothers, aunts) on the maternal side of homosexual men have more children than relatives of heterosexuals (Camperio-Ciani et al., 2004). Furthermore, this difference is not found in the paternal lineage, which is in complete agreement with the genetic studies described above that indicate that homosexuality would be inherited by genetic transmission from the mother, not the father. This study also confirmed that homosexuals have more gay relatives on the maternal than on the paternal side and that homosexuals are more frequent among younger brothers of a family than among older brothers (the older brothers effect).

The group theory of evolution (kin selection) also provides a hypothesis to explain the persistence of genes for homosexuality. Homosexual individuals who have no children themselves could help their close relatives (brothers, sisters, cousins) to raise their children who are genetically related. Under the more difficult conditions of survival that prevailed during human evolution, this additional assistance could have favored the survival of children and thus contributed to the transmission of genes promoting homosexuality. Many animal societies have been identified in which some individuals do not reproduce, but simply help raise the offspring of their close relatives. This reproduction, based on a few individuals helped by others closely related to them genetically, is almost always observed in difficult environmental conditions (e.g., deserts) and is expected to be maintained because the nonbreeding individuals still spread their genes through the reproduction of their close relatives. This seemingly altruistic behavior would be still "interested" from an evolutionary point of view.

It is also possible that genes controlling homosexuality are only harmful to reproduction and therefore have a tendency to disappear on a continuous basis. They would be maintained in humans by repeated mutations that would frequently make them reappear in a more or less similar form. Sites on the chromosomes are known that are actually subject to very frequent mutations, but so far none has been associated with homosexuality.

It is clear that as long as the gene or genes favoring homosexuality have not been identified, it remains impossible to test these different interpretations. They are presented here simply to show that the existence of a gene to a phenotypic trait obviously associated with a decreased reproductive success is not inconceivable.

11

General Conclusions

At the end of this journey into the world of neurobiology in relation to sexuality, it is important to summarize the accumulated knowledge and the questions that remain unanswered, and then see how scientific information collected over the past 20 or 30 years can and should probably change certain aspects of medical practice and also, in a much more important manner, the general attitude of society toward homosexuals (and also probably transsexuals).

WHAT CONTEMPORARY NEUROBIOLOGY TEACHES US

A dozen important points should be recalled to understand the real scope of current knowledge.

In Animals

1. The action of hormones on the hypothalamus and preoptic area in rodents and primates precisely determines the type of sexual behavior (male or female) expressed by an individual. This determination is largely independent of the genetic sex of the animal. It is controlled by the type of hormonal imprinting experienced during embryonic and/or immediately postpartum life

in interaction with the hormones that are secreted by the testes or ovaries in adulthood.

2. The embryonic sex steroids also differentiate the size of several brain structures, including the SDN-POA and, once acquired, this size is typical of one sex and cannot be changed in adulthood by steroid hormones.

3. Male sexual orientation is determined by the action of sex steroids in the preoptic area. It is modified (inverted) by hormonal treatments during early development in young animals (the same treatments that are changing the type of behaviors that will be exhibited later), and thereafter orientation seems to be a stable characteristic of the individual. This orientation can be manipulated at will by injections of steroids in a developing individual, but not in adulthood.

4. The only case of spontaneous strict homosexuality in animals is observed in sheep. Homosexual male sheep have a sexually dimorphic nucleus of the preoptic area the same size as that of a female. The size of this nucleus is determined by the action of testosterone during embryonic life.

In Humans

5. The sex steroids and their receptors in the human brain are similar or identical to what they are in animals. One can find in the human species all the embryonic effects of sex steroids on genital structures that are identified in animals. Effects of steroids are also present in the activation of sexual behavior even though they are, as might be expected given the complexity of human sexuality, more nuanced than in animals.

6. The sexual differentiation of genital structures during embryonic life precedes by several months the differentiation of the brain, the organ controlling behavior. It is therefore possible that hormonal changes occurring between these two embryonic periods can induce discrepancies between physical sex and aspects of sexual behavior that are sexually differentiated (orientation, gender identity). Such discrepancies could also originate in a differential sensitivity of responses to steroids (dose-response difference) or in the existence of different sensitive periods to the action of steroids.

7. Homosexuality is not simply a different sexual orientation; it is accompanied by complex physical, functional, and behavioral changes. Homosexuality therefore affects not only a particular aspect

of sexual behavior but also multiple sexually differentiated traits that are not related to sexuality. Male (female) homosexuality is a complex change, often in a female (male) direction, of multiple features that are sexually differentiated. These characteristics include variables that possibly could be secondarily affected by homosexuality (e.g., responses in cognitive tests) but also physical (ratio of length of fingers D2:D4) or functional (oto-acoustic emissions produced by the inner ear) variables. It is hard to see how these variables could be influenced by sexual orientation.

8. A physical difference associated with homosexuality of particular interest is the difference that affects the size of the sexually dimorphic nucleus of preoptic area (SDN-POA). It is larger in heterosexual men than in women and that of male homosexuals is the size of a female's. The mechanism that controls the development of this nucleus in humans is unknown, but it does not seem to significantly depend on the hormonal status in adulthood. In rats and sheep, the size of the nucleus is determined irreversibly by the action of embryonic sex steroids, and its lesion in adult male rats changes sexual orientation.

9. Many diseases that affect the functioning of the endocrine system during fetal life are associated with more or less profound changes of sexual orientation in men and women. In a limited number of these pathologies, children are raised as if they belonged to a sex opposed to the potential hormonal influence they have been exposed to in utero. A substantial proportion of subjects exposed to such "experiments of nature" or pseudo-experiments develop a sexual orientation (and sometimes a sexual identity) in opposition to the sex of the education they have received. This suggests an important role of embryonic hormones in determining these behavioral characteristics.

10. Various arguments, including many studies of the sexual orientation of twins, clearly indicate a genetic contribution (but not an absolute determinism) of sexual orientation. If one twin is homosexual, the probability that the second is also gay is much higher in "real" twins originating from one egg and thus sharing the same genetic material than among the "false" fraternal twins.

11. The genetic contribution to male homosexuality is apparently inherited preferentially through the maternal line. This observation led to the identification of a region of the X chromosome whose variability is significantly associated with sexual orientation. This association has been identified several times independently, but to date one or more genes linked to homosexuality still have not been

isolated. The genetic contribution to sexual orientation is most likely multigenic and therefore very difficult to identify.

12. The most reliable factor identified for the development of homosexuality in the male is the presence in his family of older brothers born to the same mother. In these circumstances, the likelihood of homosexuality increases by 33% for each older brother and is accompanied by a small but statistically significant decrease in weight at birth. These effects do not appear to be explained by differences in education or family and are presumably the result of the accumulation in the mother, during successive pregnancies, of antibodies against one or more proteins expressed specifically by boys but not yet identified.

Taken together, all these data thus strongly suggest that hormonal, genetic, and possibly immunological factors acting to a large extent during the embryonic life or during early infancy play an import role in the determination of sexual orientation.

THERE IS NO PSYCHOANALYTIC, PSYCHOLOGICAL, OR SOCIOLOGICAL EXPLANATION OF HOMOSEXUALITY

In contrast, the alternative explanations of homosexuality that are based on psychoanalysis, psychology, or sociology are perhaps attractive at first glance, but the rare quantitative studies that were conducted to test them provide, to our knowledge, no support. Psychoanalytic interpretations are mainly based on series of anecdotes related to the analysis performed by Sigmund Freud himself, whose scientific honesty was seriously questioned (Van Rillaer, 1980; Bénesteau, 2002; Dufresne, 2007).

It seems well established that the sexual and social experiences of early childhood and adolescence have little or no effect on the development of homosexuality. Theories of homosexuality derived from psychoanalysis, behaviorism, or social constructivism, attributing a major role to early sexual experiences or relationships with parents, did not find any support in controlled scientific studies and are in fact at odds with many facts of observation. For example, children raised by homosexual couples are not more likely to become homosexual than children raised by heterosexual couples. The absence of the father has no effect on the occurrence of male homosexuality (no increase among children raised by a single mother), and the frequency of homosexuality is not larger (it is in fact similar in all human societies) in some societies in New Guinea, where homosexual experiences are the rule among the adolescent boys, or in boys who have been raised in boarding schools where homosexual relations were present on a regular basis during adolescence.

These negative results do not necessarily imply the complete absence of influence of the postnatal environment on the development of sexual orientation, but available data strongly suggest that the environment alone cannot determine homosexuality or heterosexuality, though it is quite conceivable that it may interact with prenatal biological factors that I have outlined to allow their full expression. Studies that could potentially identify such interactions should probably be based on extremely large numbers of subjects, given the low amplitude of the effects studied.

WHAT ARE THE KEY POINTS THAT SHOULD BE REMEMBERED?

Even taking into account the limitations described in earlier chapters, it seems undeniable that the balance between biological and cultural factors that may explain homosexuality very much favors the biological factors acting predominantly during embryonic life. Human (and animal) homosexuality is the result of an interaction between hormonal and genetic embryonic factors with perhaps a minor contribution of postnatal social and sexual experiences.

Studies on twins show a significant genetic contribution that could explain at least 50% of the variance in sexual orientation in Western societies. Various prenatal endocrine disorders affect orientation, but in no known case is there is percentage of induced homosexuality greater than about 30%. Finally, the observed associations between homosexuality and the modification of sexually differentiated characteristics are often statistically significant, but they are also related to a definite level of variability. Taking the size of the SDN of the preoptic area once again as an example, this nucleus is twice smaller on average in homosexuals than in heterosexuals. However, at the individual level there are heterosexuals who have an SDN whose size is close to the gay average, and conversely there are homosexuals who have a relatively large SDN that therefore falls within the normal distribution for heterosexuals. The association between size of the SDN and sexual orientation is statistically validated, but it does not apply for each individual.

It is thus clear that none of the biological factors identified to date is able by itself to explain homosexuality. Three potential explanations are therefore possible. Either there are different types of homosexuality—some have a genetic origin, others a hormonal origin, still others result from the older brothers effect or from biological factors not yet identified—or the effects of different biological factors that have been identified interact with each other in a variable manner in each individual and it is only when several of these predisposing factors are combined that homosexual orientation is observed, or finally, all the biological factors that I have described only produce a predisposition to become homosexual, and these predispositions can only develop in a specific set of psychosocial contexts that are not yet identified. But if this postnatal context is actually an important permissive factor, it is surprising that a quantitative study has been unable so far to identify aspects of the environment that are limiting.

Current knowledge does not allow us to discriminate between these interpretations. However, it is clear that biological factors acting during prenatal life play a significant role in determining sexual orientation and that homosexuality is not, for most people, a choice of life. This orientation is often or always an evidence that imposes itself on the individual during his or her teens or life as a young adult. The recognition of a nonconventional sexual orientation is very often the occasion of significant psychological suffering. Remember the suicide rate that is three times higher during adolescence among homosexuals as compared to the general population. By contrast, the heterosexual orientation develops spontaneously, often while the individual does not truly realize it. It is not a matter of choice here. One does not choose to be homosexual any more than one chooses to be heterosexual. We can choose to accept this orientation, to act accordingly, and to reveal it or not to the society, but the orientation itself is not in any way a deliberate choice. Given the complexity of the human person, this does not mean of course that there is not a minority of gay men for whom this sexual orientation is a choice of life influenced by past experiences and/or motivated by various reasons ranging from curiosity to perversity.

There are probably sex perverts among homosexuals, just as there are among heterosexuals, but homosexuality itself is not a perversion. A large proportion of homosexuals are born with that sexual orientation, which is revealed to them in a very progressive way during development and is often accepted at the price of a significant psychological distress. It is for most of them not a choice (how could a homosexual change by personal choice his D2:D4 ratio or the functioning of his or her inner ear?). Homosexuality is due neither to a perversity nor to inadequate parents. It is a biological variation of a complex behavioral trait whose control is obviously multifactorial.

WHAT ARE THE CONSEQUENCES?

It was thought for a long time that the young child is a tabula rasa and that it is possible through education to impose a sexual identity and sexual orientation independent of the genetic sex (Money & Ehrhardt, 1972). The exemplary case of John/Joan and many other studies that were reviewed clearly suggest that this is not the case and that sexual identity and sexual orientation are, at least in part, determined before birth. The clearest demonstration of this prenatal control is provided by the occurrence of cloacal exstrophy. It seems that the hormonal embryonic imprinting or possibly the genetic sex itself have an influence on gender identity and sexual orientation. The results of animal experiments associated with correlations derived from human clinical data thus suggest that people are born gay, they do not become homosexual, contrary to a widespread idea. This finding has important implications in two quite different areas.

UNDERSTANDING DOES NOT MEAN ACTING: THE EUGENIC RISK

It is important to clarify that the purpose of science in general and this book in particular is not to identify the biological mechanisms that control the emergence of homosexuality in order to control this aspect of human sexuality. The goal here is simply to understand the functioning of the animal and human brain and advance the objective knowledge of human nature. I believe that a better understanding of the mechanisms that control sexual orientation (homosexual as well as heterosexual) should have positive effects on how society views homosexuals and should help their parents understand that they are not responsible for the sexual orientation of their child.

At the same time we must not ignore the consequences of this research and we must seriously ask ourselves whether knowledge of these mechanisms would be likely to lead to eugenic abuses, which could either propose abortion of embryos for which there is a increased risk of homosexuality or in the future propose treatment that would potentially change this prenatal predisposition. This risk is of course present as soon as a society is exposed to ethical drifts and no longer controls the use of its science and technology. Several remarks are in order at this level, however.

First, it should be noted that even if we now have converging information strongly supporting the idea that homosexuality is controlled by prenatal hormonal and/or genetic factors, we are still far from understanding the details of these mechanisms to thus be able to modify these processes to obtain a specific result. It is likely that this relative ignorance will persist for many years and we will therefore not be able to "choose" the desired sexual orientation for a future child.

Furthermore, for ethically deviant societies (e.g., Nazi or communist countries), an understanding of the determinism of homosexuality is not necessary and was not necessary in the past to persecute homosexuals and even sometimes condemn them to death. That is still the case in countries such as Iran or Afghanistan. Societies as well as social, religious, or medical groups who want to hurt homosexuals do not need to understand the mechanisms that control this sexual orientation to combat homosexuality. Their ignorance is sufficient, and if the truth is likely to prevent the deeds of such extremist groups, it cannot support them.

It also should be noted that understanding does not necessarily mean wanting to control. Understanding is part of science; the choice of the use of knowledge is a question of morality and politics. It is very important that scientists be involved in the political choices that are made, particularly when they concern the use of science and technology, but the two aspects of human activity should not be confused. It would be foolish to abandon the pursuit of knowledge because it could later be misused. If this were the case, then we would have had to abandon the discovery of the structure of the atom. This knowledge has brought significant benefits (radiotherapy, an enormous source of energy) as well as major disasters (the atomic bomb). It is up to societies to decide what they do with scientific knowledge. In our view, understanding the biological mechanisms that control human behavior should have more positive than negative effects on the happiness of the human species.

THE ATTITUDE OF SOCIETY TOWARD HOMOSEXUALS SHOULD (STILL) CHANGE

Throughout history, homosexuals have been persecuted for many reasons and homosexuality was considered a sin, a disease, or a perversion. This type of opinion has changed during the 20th century, at least for a large number of people in Europe and the United States. In these countries many homosexuals are now free to display their sexual orientation, even to marry and adopt children. However, the fact remains that this sexual orientation is often difficult to assume and is associated in the mind of many people, even those with a high degree of education, with notions of deviance, perversion, and guilt. Many parents are also affected by a deep sense of guilt because they mistakenly think they somehow should have provided different conditions for a "normal" development of their child.

Biological studies presented in this work, even though they do not identify the mechanisms that lead to homosexuality in a formal manner, nonetheless clearly show that homosexuality is not, in general, a free choice of life and that any role of parents in its appearance can be only very marginal and may not even exist at all. The fact that homosexuality is statistically associated with physical (the D2:D4 ratio of finger sizes) or functional (oto-acoustic emissions) differences shows that this is not a choice. Homosexuality should therefore be regarded as a spontaneous variation of a biological character. This character (sexual orientation) and its determinism are complex, but there is no reason to believe a priori that the status of this character is different from that of any other physical/functional trait such as height or hair color. Just as one does not choose to be left-handed or right-handed, one cannot choose to be homosexual or heterosexual.

Finally, we must recognize that there are homosexuals who claim their lifestyle and say, contrary to the argument presented in this book, that their sexual orientation reflects a free choice of life. I respect this attitude and give everyone the right to do what he or she wants with the data presented here. The level of biological determinism that has been identified to date remains imprecise and can leave a place for individual choice. Large interindividual variations in the determinism of homosexuality probably exist and homosexuality is not, in all probability, a uniform phenomenon. If some think that they are homosexual by choice, there is no reason to try to dissuade them, and it is possible that they are right. In many other cases, however, homosexuality is seen as a "defect" or a perversion that is in conflict with deep religious or moral convictions. For many homosexuals, homosexuality was never an option but a difference difficult to accept and a challenge for social integration. To all these people, we should be able to say that the difference is essentially the same as the difference that affects people in relation to their stature, eye color, or hair color. Determinism of sexual orientation is simply more complex than that of these physical characteristics.

If we accept these premises, it becomes apparent that homosexuals and their parents are not responsible for their sexual orientation and there is no objective reason to reject them. Homosexuals are not perverse (at least not more than straight people), they are not dangerous (homosexuality is not "contagious"), and they are generally not responsible for their condition. They should be able to live their lives according to their nature (biology) without worrying about issues of personal guilt. In return, society should, as it is increasingly but not yet uniformly doing, accept them without any form of discrimination.

REFERENCES

Abdelgadir, S.E., Roselli, C.E., Choate, J.V. & Resko, J.A. (1999) Androgen receptor messenger ribonucleic acid in brains and pituitaries of male rhesus monkeys: studies on distribution, hormonal control, and relationship to luteinizing hormone secretion. *Biol Reprod*, **60**, 1251–1256.

Adkins-Regan, E. (1999) Testosterone increases singing and aggression but not male-typical sexual partner preference in early estrogen treated female zebra finches. *Horm. Behav.*, **35**, 63–70.

Adkins-Regan, E. (2011) Neuroendocrine contributions to sexual partner preference in birds. *Front Neuroendocrinol*, **32**, 155–163.

Adkins-Regan, E. & Ascenzi, M. (1987) Social and sexual behaviour of male and female zebra finches treated with oestradiol during the nestling period. *Anim. Behav.*, **35**, 1100–1112.

Adkins-Regan, E. & Wade, J. (2001) Masculinized sexual partner preference in female zebra finches with sex-reversed gonads. *Horm. Behav.*, **39**, 22–28.

Adkins-Regan, E., Yang, S. & Mansukhani, V. (1996) Behavior of male and female zebra finches treated with an estrogen synthesis inhibitor as nestlings. *Behaviour*, **133**, 847–862.

Agmo, A. (2007) *Functional and dysfunctional sexual behavior. A synthesis of neuroscience and comparative psychology.* Elsevier, Amsterdam.

Ahmed, E.I., Zehr, J.L., Schulz, K.M., Lorenz, B.H., DonCarlos, L.L. & Sisk, C.L. (2008) Pubertal hormones modulate the addition of new cells to sexually dimorphic brain regions. *Nat. Neurosci.*, **11**, 995–997.

Alexander, B.M., Rose, J.D., Stellflug, J.N., Fitzgerald, J.A. & Moss, G.E. (1999) Behavior and endocrine changes in high-performing, low-performing, and male-oriented domestic rams following exposure to rams and ewes in estrus when copulation is precluded. *J. Anim. Sci.*, **77**, 1869–1874.

Alexander, G.M. & Hines, M. (2002) Sex diferences in response to children's toys in non-human primates (Cercopithecus aethios sabaeus). *Evolution and Human Behavior*, **23**, 467–479.

Allen, L.S. & Gorski, R.A. (1992) Sexual orientation and the size of the anterior commissure in the human brain. *Proc. Natl. Acad. Sci. USA*, **89**, 7199–7202.

Allen, L.S., Hines, M., Shryne, J.E. & Gorski, R.A. (1989) Two sexually dimorphic cell groups in the human brain. *J. Neurosci*, **9**, 497–506.

Anderson, D.K., Rhees, R.W. & Fleming, D.E. (1985) Effects of prenatal stress on differentiation of the sexually dimorphic nucleus of the preoptic area (SDN-POA) of the rat brain. *Brain Res.*, **332**, 113–118.

Arnold, A.P. & Chen, X. (2009) What does the "four core genotypes" mouse model tell us about sex differences in the brain and other tissues? *Front Neuroendocrinol*, **30**, 1–9.

Arnold, A.P. & Gorski, R.A. (1984) Gonadal steroid induction of structural sex differences in the central nervous system. *Ann. Rev. Neurosci.*, **7**, 413–442.

Arnold, A.P., Xu, J., Grisham, W., Chen, X.Q., Kim, Y.H. & Itoh, Y. (2004) Minireview: Sex chromosomes and brain sexual differentiation. *Endocrinology*, **145**, 1057–1062.

Bagatell, C.J., Heiman, J.R., Rivier, J.E. & Bremner, W.J. (1994) Effects of endogenous testosterone and estradiol on sexual behavior in normal young men. *J. Clin. Endocrinol. Metab.*, **78**, 711–716.

Bagemihl, B. (1999) *Biological exuberance. Animal homosexuality and natural diversity.* St. Martin's Press, New York.

Bailey, J.M., Willerman, L. & Parks, C. (1991) A test of the maternal stress theory of human male homosexuality. *Arch Sex. Behav.*, **20**, 277–293.

Bakker, J., Baum, M.J. & Slob, A.K. (1996a) Neonatal inhibition of brain estrogen synthesis alters adult neural Fos responses to mating and pheromonal stimulation in the male rat. *Neuroscience*, **74**, 251–260.

Bakker, J., Brand, T., van Ophemert, J. & Slob, A.K. (1993a) Hormonal regulation of adult partner preference behavior in neonatally ATD-treated male rats. *Behav. Neurosci.*, **107**, 480–487.

Bakker, J. & Brock, O. (2010) Early oestrogens in shaping reproductive networks: evidence for a potential organisational role of oestradiol in female brain development. *J. Neuroendocrinol*, **22**, 728–735.

Bakker, J., De Mees, C., Douhard, Q., Balthazart, J., Gabant, P., Szpirer, J. & Szpirer, C. (2006) Alpha-fetoprotein protects the developing female mouse brain from masculinization and defeminization by estrogens. *Nat Neurosci.*, **9**, 220–226.

Bakker, J., Honda, S., Harada, N. & Balthazart, J. (2002a) Sexual partner preference requires a functional aromatase (cyp19) gene in male mice. *Horm. Behav.*, **42**, 158–171.

Bakker, J., Honda, S.I., Harada, N. & Balthazart, J. (2002b) The aromatase knock-out mouse provides new evidence that estradiol is required during development in the female for the expression of sociosexual behaviors in adulthood. *J. Neurosci.*, **22**, 9104–9112.

Bakker, J., Van Ophemert, J. & Slob, A.K. (1993b) Organization of partner preference and sexual behavior and its nocturnal rhythmicity in male rats. *Behav. Neurosci.*, **107**, 1049–1058.

Bakker, J., Van Ophemert, J. & Slob, A.K. (1996b) Sexual differentiation of odor and partner preference in the rat. *Physiol. Behav.*, **60**, 489–494.

Balthazart, J. & Ball, G.F. (2006) Is brain estradiol a hormone or a neurotransmitter? *Trends Neurosci.*, **29**, 241–249.

Balthazart, J. & Ball, G.F. (2007) Topography in the preoptic region: differential regulation of appetitive and consummatory male sexual behaviors. *Front Neuroendocrinol*, **28**, 161–178.

Balthazart, J., Cornil, C.A., Charlier, T.D., Taziaux, M. & Ball, G.F. (2009) Estradiol, a key endocrine signal in the sexual differentiation and activation of reproductive behavior in quail. *J Exp Zool Part A Ecol Genet Physiol*. **311**, 323–345.

Bancroft, J. (1995) *The pharmacology of sexual function and dysfunction*. Elsevier Science, Amsterdam.

Baron-Cohen, S. (2004) *The Essential Difference: Men, Women and the Extreme Male Brain*. Penguin Press Science, London.

Baron-Cohen, S. (2006) *Prenatal testosterone in mind*. MIT Press, Cambridge, MA.

Barres., B.A. (2010) Neuro Nonsense. *Plos Biology*, **8**, e1001005.

Baum, M.J., Carroll, R.S., Erskine, M.S. & Tobet, S.A. (1985) Neuroendocrine response to estrogen and sexual orientation. *Science*, 230, 960–961.

Becker, J.B., Berkley, K.J., Geary, N., Hampson, E., Herman, J.P. & Young, E.A. (2008) *Sex differences in the brain. From Genes to behavior*. Oxford University Press, Oxford.

Becker, J.B., Breedlove, S.M., Crews, D. & McCarthy, M.M. (2002) *Behavioral Endocrinology*. MIT Press, Cambridge MA.

Bell, A.P., Weinberg, M.S. & Hammersmith, S.K. (1981) *Sexual preference: It's development in men and women*. Indiana University Press, Bloomington.

Benbow, C.P. (1993) Sex differences in mathematical reasoning ability in intellectually talented preadolescents: Their nature, effects and possible causes. BBS 11:169–232. *Behav. Brain Sci.*, **16**, 187–189.

Bénesteau, J. (2002) *Mensonges Freudiens*. Pierre Mardaga, Wavre (Belgique).

Berenbaum, S.A., Bryk, K.K., Nowak, N., Quigley, C.A. & Moffat, S. (2009) Fingers as a marker of prenatal androgen exposure. *Endocrinology*, **150**, 5119–5124.

Berenbaum, S.A., Duck, S.C. & Bryk, K. (2000) Behavioral effects of prenatal versus postnatal androgen excess in children with 21-hydroxylase-deficient congenital adrenal hyperplasia. *J Clin Endocrinol Metab*, **85**, 727–733.

Berenbaum, S.A. & Hines, M. (1992) Early androgens are related to childhood sex-typed toy preferences. *Psychol. Sci.*, **3**, 203–206.

Berenbaum, S.A. & Snyder, E. (1995) Early hormonal influences on childhood sex-typed activity and playmate preferences: implications for the development of sexual orientation. *Developmental Psychology*, **31**, 31–42.

Berglund, H., Lindstrom, P. & Savic, I. (2006) Brain response to putative pheromones in lesbian women. *Proc. Natl. Acad. Sci. U S A*, **103**, 8269–8274.

Berta, P., Hawkins, J.R., Sinclair, A.H., Taylor, A., Griffiths, B.L., Goodfellow, P.N. & Fellous, M. (1990) Genetic evidence equating SRY and the testis-determining factor. *Nature*, **348**, 448–450.

Berthold, A.A. (1849) Transplantation der Hoden. *Arch. F. Anat. U. Physiol.*, **16**, 42–46.

Blanchard, R. (1997) Birth order and sibling sex ration in homosexual versus heterosexual males and females. *Ann. Rev. Sex Res.* **8**, 27–67.

Blanchard, R. (2001) Fraternal birth order and the maternal immune hypothesis of male homosexuality. *Horm. Behav.*, **40**, 105–114.

Blanchard, R. (2004) Quantitative and theoretical analyses of the relation between older brothers and homosexuality in men. *J. Theor. Biol.* 230, 173–187.

Blanchard, R. & Bogaert, A.F. (1996) Homosexuality in men and number of older brothers. *Am. J. Psychiatry*, **153**, 27–31.

Blanchard, R., Cantor, J.M., Bogaert, A.F., Breedlove, S.M. & Ellis, L. (2006) Interaction of fraternal birth order and handedness in the development of male homosexuality. *Horm. Behav.*, **49**, 405–414.

Blanchard, R. & Klassen, P. (1997) H-Y antigen and homosexuality in men. *J. Theor. Biol.*, **185**, 373–378.

Blanchard, R. & Lippa, R.A. (2007) Birth order, sibling sex ratio, handedness, and sexual orientation of male and female participants in a BBC internet research project. *Arch. Sex. Behav.*, **36**, 163–176.

Bloch, G.J. & Gorski, R.A. (1988a) Cytoarchitectonic analysis of the SDN-POA of the intact and gonadectomized rat. *J. Comp. Neurol.*, **275**, 604–612.

Bloch, G.J. & Gorski, R.A. (1988b) Estrogen/progesterone treatment in adulthood affects the size of several components of the medial preoptic area in the male rat. *J. Comp. Neurol.*, **275**, 613–622.

Bocklandt, S., Horvath, S., Vilain, E. & Hamer, D.H. (2006) Extreme skewing of X chromosome inactivation in mothers of homosexual men. *Hum. Genet.*, **118**, 691–694.

Bocklandt, S. & Vilain, E. (2007) Sex differences in brain and behavior: hormones versus genes. *Adv. Genet.*, **59**, 245–266.

Bodo, C. & Rissman, E.F. (2007) Androgen receptor is essential for sexual differentiation of responses to olfactory cues in mice. *Eur. J. Neurosci.*, **25**, 2182–2190.

Bodo, C. & Rissman, E.F. (2008) The androgen receptor is selectively involved in organization of sexually dimorphic social behaviors in mice. *Endocrinology*, **149**, 4142–4150.

Bogaert, A.F. (2006) Biological versus nonbiological older brothers and men's sexual orientation. *Proc. Natl. Acad. Sci. U S A*, **103**, 10771–10774.

Bogaert, A.F. & Skorska, M. (2011) Sexual Orientation, Fraternal Birth Order, and the Maternal Immune Hypothesis: A Review of Evidence. *Front Neuroendocrinol*, **32**, 247–254.

Bradley, S.J., Oliver, G.D., Chernick, A.B. & Zucker, K.J. (1998) Experiment of nurture: ablatio penis at 2 months, sex reassignment at 7 months, and a psychosexual follow-up in young adulthood. *Pediatrics*, **102**, 1–5.

Breedlove, S.M. (2010) Minireview: Organizational hypothesis: instances of the fingerpost. *Endocrinology*, **151**, 4116–4122.

Brock, O. & Bakker, J. (2011) Potential contribution of prenatal estrogens to the sexual differentiation of mate preferences in mice. *Horm. Behav.*, **59**, 83–89.

Brown, W.M., Finn, C.J., Cooke, B.M. & Breedlove, S.M. (2002a) Differences in finger length ratios between self-identified "butch" and "femme" lesbians. *Arch. Sex. Behav.*, **31**, 123–127.

Brown, W.M., Hines, M., Fane, B.A. & Breedlove, S.M. (2002b) Masculinized finger length patterns in human males and females with congenital adrenal hyperplasia. *Horm. Behav.*, **42**, 380–386.

Byne, W., Tobet, S., Mattiace, L.A., Lasco, M.S., Kemether, E., Edgar, M.A., Morgello, S., Buchsbaum, M.S. & Jones, L.B. (2001) The interstitial nuclei of the human anterior hypothalamus: An investigation of variation with sex, sexual orientation, and HIV status. *Horm. Behav.*, **40**, 86–92.

Cameron, P. & Cameron, K. (1995) Does incest cause homosexuality? *Psychol. Rep.*, **76**, 611–621.

Campbell, B.C., Prossinger, H. & Mbzivo, M. (2005) Timing of Pubertal Maturation and the Onset of Sexual Behavior among Zimbabwe School Boys. *Arch. Sexual Behav.*, **34**, 505–516.

Camperio-Ciani, A., Corna, F. & Capiluppi, C. (2004) Evidence for maternally inherited factors favouring male homosexuality and promoting female fecundity. *Proc. Biol. Sci*, **271**, 2217–2221.

Carani, C., Bancroft, J., Granata, A., Del Rio, G. & Marrama, P. (1992) Testosterone and erectile function, nocturnal penile tumescence and rigidity, and erectile response to visual erotic stimuli in hypogonadal and eugonadal men. *Psychoneuroendocrinology*, **17**, 647–654.

Carani, C., Granata, A.R., Rochira, V., Caffagni, G., Aranda, C., Antunez, P. & Maffei, L.E. (2005) Sex steroids and sexual desire in a man with a novel mutation of aromatase gene and hypogonadism. *Psychoneuroendocrinology*, **30**, 413–417.

Carani, C., Rochira, V., Faustini-Fustini, M., Balestrieri, A. & Granata, A.R.M. (1999) Role of oestrogen in male sexual behaviour: insights from the natural model of aromatase deficiency. *Clinical Endocrinology*, **51**, 517–524.

Chivers, M.L., Rieger, G., Latty, E. & Bailey, J.M. (2004) A sex difference in the specificity of sexual arousal. *Psychol. Sci.*, **15**, 736–744.

Chung, W.C.J., De Vries, G.J. & Swaab, D.F. (2002) Sexual differentiation of the bed nucleus of the stria terminalis in humans may extend into adulthood. *J. Neurosci.*, **22**, 1027–1033.

Churchill, W. (1967) *Homosexual behavior among males: A cross-cultural and cross-species investigation*. Hawthorn books, New York.

Colapinto, J. (2000) **As nature made him: The boy that was raised as a girl**. Harper Collins, New York.

Collaer, M.L. & Hines, M. (1995) Human behavioral sex differences: a role for gonadal hormones during early development? *Psychol. Bull.*, **118**, 55–107.

Connellan, J., Baron-Cohen, S., Wheelwright, S., Batk, A. & Ahluwalia, J. (2000) Sex differences in human neonatal social perception. *Infant Behav. Develop*, **23**, 113–118.

Cooke, B.M., Tabibnia, G. & Breedlove, S.M. (1999) A brain sexual dimorphism controlled by adult circulating androgens. *Proc. Natl. Acad. Sci. USA*, **96**, 7538–7540.

Cooper, J.R., Bloom, F.E. & Roth, R.H. (1996) *The biochemical basis of neuropharmacology*. Oxford University Press, New York.

Cornil, C.A., Ball, G.F. & Balthazart, J. (2006) Functional significance of the rapid regulation of brain estrogen action: Where do the estrogens come from? *Brain Res.*, **1126**, 2–26.

Crews, D., Camazine, B., Diamond, M., Mason, R., Tokarz, R. & Gartska, W.R. (1984) Hormonal independence of courtship behavior in the male garter snake. *Horm. Behav.*, **18**, 29–41.

Crews, D. & Gartska, W.R. (1982) The ecological physiology of a garter snake. *Sci. Am.*, **247**, 159–168.

Davidson, J.M., Camargo, C.A. & Smith, E.R. (1979) Effects of androgen on sexual behavior in hypogonadal men. *J. Clin. Endocrinol. Metab.*, **48**, 955–958.

Davis, E.C., Shryne, J.E. & Gorski, R.A. (1995) A revised critical period for the sexual differentiation of the sexually dimorphic nucleus of the preoptic area in the rat. *Neuroendocrinol.*, **62**, 579–585.

de Lacoste-Utamsing, C. & Holloway, R.L. (1982) Sexual dimorphism in the human corpus callosum. *Science*, **216**, 1431–1432.

De Vries, G.J., Rissman, E.F., Simerly, R.B., Yang, L.Y., Scordalakes, E.M., Auger, C.J., Swain, A., Lovell-Badge, R., Burgoyne, P.S. & Arnold, A.P. (2002) A model system for study of sex chromosome effects on sexually dimorphic neural and behavioral traits. *J. Neurosci.*, **22**, 9005–9014.

Diamond, M. (1993) Some genetic considerations in the development of sexual orientation. In Haug, M., Whalen, R.E., Aron, C., Olsen, K.L. (eds) *The development of sex differences and similarities in behavior*. Kluwer Academic Publishers, Dordrecht, pp. 291–309.

Diamond, M. & Sigmundson, H.K. (1997) Sex reassignment at birth: long-term review and clinical implications. *Arch. Pediatrics and Adolescent Medicine*, **151**, 298–304.

Dittmann, R.W., Kappes, M.E. & Kappes, M.H. (1992) Sexual behavior in adolescent and adult females with congenital adrenal hyperplasia. *Psychoneuroendocrinology*, **17**, 153–170.

Dörner, G. (1969) Zur Frage einer neuroendocrinen Pathogenese, Prophylaxe und Therapie angeborenen Sexualdeviationen. *Deutsche Medizinische Wochenschrift*, **94**, 390–396.

Dörner, G. (1972) *Sexualhormonabhängige Gehirndifferenzierung und Sexualität*. Springer, Berlin, Heidelberg, New York.

Dörner, G. (1976) *Hormones and Brain Differentiation*. Elsevier, Amsterdam, Oxford, New York.

Dörner, G. (1980) Sexual differentiation of the brain *Vitamins and hormones*. Academic Press, Inc., pp. 325–381, New York.

Dörner, G., Geier, T., Ahrens, L., Krell, L., Munx, G., Sieler, H., Kittner, E. & Muller, H. (1980) Prenatal stress as possible aetiogenetic factor of homosexuality in human males. *Endokrinologie*, **75**, 365–368.

Dörner, G., Schenk, B., Schmiedel, B. & Ahrens, L. (1983) Stressful events in prenatal life of bi- and homosexual men. *Exp Clin Endocrinol*, **81**, 83–87.

Dörner, G. & Staudt, J. (1969) Structural changes in the hypothalamic ventromedial nucleus of the male rat, following neonatal castration and androgen treatment. *Neuroendocrinol.*, **4**, 278–281.

Dubb, A., Gur, R., Avants, B. & Gee, J. (2003) Characterization of sexual dimorphism in the human corpus callosum. *Neuroimage*, **20**, 512–519.

Dufresne, T. (2007) *Against Freud. Critics talk back*. Stanford University Press, Stanford, CA.

Ehrhardt, A.A., Meyer-Bahlburg, H.F., Rosen, L.R., Feldman, J.F., Veridiano, N.P., Zimmerman, I. & McEwen, B.S. (1985) Sexual orientation after prenatal exposure to exogenous estrogen. *Arch. Sex. Behav.*, **14**, 57–77.

Elbert, T., Pantev, C., Wienbruch, C., Rockstroh, B. & Taub, E. (1995) Increased cortical representation of the fingers of the left hand in string players. *Science*, **270**, 305–307.

Ellis, L., Ames, M.A., Peckham, W. & Ahrens, L. (1988) Sexual orientation of human offspring may be altered by severe maternal stress during pregnancy. *J. Sex. Res.*, **25**, 152–157.

Ellis, L., Hershberger, S., Field, E., Wersinger, S., Pelis, S., Geary, D., Palmer, C., Hoyenga, K., Hetsroni, A. & Karadi, K. (2008) *Sex differences: summarizing more than a century of scientific research.* Psychology Press, New York.

Ellis, L., Hoffman, H. & Burke, D.M. (1990) Sex, sexual orientation and criminal and violent behavior. *Personality and Individual Differences*, **11**, 1207–1211.

Everitt, B.J. (1990) Sexual motivation: a neural and behavioural analysis of the mechanisms underlying appetitive and copulatory responses in male rats. *Neurosci. Biobehav. Rev.*, **14**, 217–232.

Everitt, B.J. (1995) Neuroendocrine mechanisms underlying appetitive and consummatory elements of masculine sexual behavior. In Bancroft, J. (ed) *The pharmacology of sexual function and dysfunction.* Elsevier, Amsterdam, pp. 15–31.

Fernández-Guasti, A., Kruijver, F.P., Fodor, M. & Swaab, D.F. (2000) Sex differences in the distribution of androgen receptors in the human hypothalamus. *J. Comp. Neurol.*, **425**, 422–435.

Fine, C. (2010) *Delusions of gender: how our minds, society and neurosexism create difference.* W.W. Norton and Company, New York.

Foidart, A., Legros, J.J. & Balthazart, J. (1994) Les phéromones humaines: vestige animal ou réalité non reconnue. *Revue Médicale de Liège*, **49**, 662–680.

Fraga, M.F., Ballestar, E., Paz, M.F., Ropero, S., Setien, F., Ballestar, M.L., Heine-Suner, D., Cigudosa, J.C., Urioste, M., Benitez, J., Boix-Chornet, M., Sanchez-Aguilera, A., Ling, C., Carlsson, E., Poulsen, P., Vaag, A., Stephan, Z., Spector, T.D., Wu, Y.Z., Plass, C. & Esteller, M. (2005) Epigenetic differences arise during the lifetime of monozygotic twins. *Proc. Natl. Acad. Sci. U S A*, **102**, 10604–10609.

Freund, K. & Blanchard, R. (1983) Is the distant relationship of fathers and homosexual sons related to the son's erotic preference for male partners, or to the sons' atypical gender identity, or both? *Journal of Homosexuality*, **9**, 7–25.

Freund, K.W. (1974) Male homosexuality: an analysis of the pattern. In Lorraine, J.A. (ed) *Understanding homosexuality: its biological and psychological bases.* Elsevier, Amsterdam, pp. 25–81.

Garcia-Falgueras, A. & Swaab, D.F. (2008) A sex difference in the hypothalamic uncinate nucleus: relationship to gender identity. *Brain*, **131**, 3132–3146.

Gladue, B.A. (1985) Neuroendocrine response to estrogen and sexual orientation. *Science*, **230**, 961.

Gladue, B.A. & Bailey, J.M. (1995) Aggressiveness, competitiveness, and human sexual orientation. *Psychoneuroendocrinol.*, **20**, 475.

Gladue, B.A., Beatty, W.W., Larson, J. & Staton, R.D. (1990) Sexual orientation and spatial ability in men and women. *Psychobiol.*, **18**, 101–108.

Gladue, B.A., Green, R. & Hellman, R.E. (1984) Neuroendocrine response to estrogen and sexual orientation. *Science*, **225**, 1496–1499.

Gobrogge, K.L., Breedlove, S.M. & Klump, K.L. (2008) Genetic and environmental influences on 2D:4D finger length ratios: a study of monozygotic and dizygotic male and female twins. *Arch. Sex. Behav.*, **37**, 112–118.

Gorski, R.A. (1984) Critical role of the medial preoptic area in the sexual differentiation of the brain. In De Vries, G.J., De Bruin, J.P.C., Uylings, H.B.M., Corner, M.A. (eds) *Sex differences in the brain.* Elsevier, Amsterdam, pp. 129–146.

Gorski, R.A., Gordon, J.H., Shryne, J.E. & Southam, A.M. (1978) Evidence for a morphological sex difference within the medial preoptic area of the rat brain. *Brain Res.,* **148**, 333–346.

Goy, R.W. & McEwen, B.S. (1980) *Sexual differentiation of the brain.* The MIT Press, Cambridge, MA.

Green, R. (1978) Sexual identity of 37 children raised by homosexual or transsexual parents. *Am. J. Psychiatry,* **135**, 692–697.

Grimbos, T., Dawood, K., Burriss, R.P., Zucker, K.J. & Puts, D.A. (2010) Sexual orientation and the second to fourth finger length ratio: a meta-analysis in men and women. *Behav. Neurosci.,* **124**, 278–287.

Guiso, L., Monte, F., Sapienza, P. & Zingales, L. (2008) Diversity. Culture, gender, and math. *Science,* **320**, 1164–1165.

Hajjar, R.R., Kaiser, F.E. & Morley, J.E. (1997) Outcomes of long-term testosterone replacement in older hypogonadal males: a retrospective analysis. *J. Clin. Endocrinol Metab.,* **82**, 3793–3796.

Hall, L.S. & Kimura, D. (1995) Sexual orientation and performance on sexually dimorphic motor tasks. *Arch. Sex. Behav.,* **24**, 395–407.

Hall, L.S. & Love, C.T. (2003) Finger-length ratios in female monozygotic twins discordant for sexual orientation. *Arch. Sex. Behav.,* **32**, 23–28.

Halperin, D.M. (1990) *One hundred years of homosexuality and other essays on Greek love.* Routledge, New York.

Halpern, C.T., Udry, J.R. & Suchindran, C. (1998) Monthly measures of salivary testosterone predict sexual activity in adolescent males. *Archives of Sexual Behavior,* **27**, 445–465.

Halpern, C.T., Udry, R. & Suchindran, C. (1997) Testosterone Predicts Initiation of Coitus in Adolescent Females. *Psychosomatic Medicine,* **59**, 161–171.

Halpern, M. & Martinez-Marcos, A. (2003) Structure and function of the vomeronasal system: an update. *Prog Neurobiol,* **70**, 245–318.

Hamer, D.H., Hu, S., Magnuson, V.L., Hu, N. & Pattatucci, A.M.L. (1993) A linkage between DNA markers on the X chromosome and male sexual orientation. *Science,* **261**, 321–327.

Hassett, J.M., Siebert, E.R. & Wallen, K. (2008) Sex differences in rhesus monkey toy preferences parallel those of children. *Horm. Behav.,* **54**, 359–364.

Hefez, S. (2007) *Dans le coeur des hommes.* Hachette, Paris.

Henley, C.L., Nunez, A.A. & Clemens, L.G. (2009) Estrogen treatment during development alters adult partner preference and reproductive behavior in female laboratory rats. *Horm. Behav.,* **55**, 68–75.

Henley, C.L., Nunez, A.A. & Clemens, L.G. (2011) Hormones of choice: the neuroendocrinology of sexual orientation in animals. *Front Neuroendocrinol,* **32**, 146–154.

Hepper, P.G., Shahidullah, S. & White, R. (1991) Handedness in the human fetus. *Neuropsychologia,* **29**, 1107–1111.

Hines, M. (2003) Sex steroids and human behavior: prenatal androgen exposure and sex-typical play behavior in children. *Ann. N. Y. Acad. Sci.,* **1007**, 272–282.

Hines, M. (2004) *Brain gender*. Oxford University Press, Oxford.

Hines, M. (2006) Prenatal testosterone and gender-related behaviour. *Eur. J. Endocrinol.*, **155** Suppl 1, S115–121.

Hines, M. & Alexander, G.M. (2008) Monkeys, girls, boys and toys: a confirmation. Letter regarding "Sex differences in toy preferences: striking parallels between monkeys and humans." *Horm. Behav.*, **54**, 478–479; author reply 80–71.

Hines, M., Brook, C. & Conway, G.S. (2004) Androgen and psychosexual development: core gender identity, sexual orientation and recalled childhood gender role behavior in women and men with congenital adrenal hyperplasia (CAH). *J. Sex. Res.*, **41**, 75–81.

Hines, M., Fane, B.A., Pasterski, V.L., Mathews, G.A., Conway, G.S. & Brook, C. (2003) Spatial abilities following prenatal androgen abnormality: targeting and mental rotations performance in individuals with congenital adrenal hyperplasia. *Psychoneuroendocrinology*, **28**, 1010–1026.

Hines, M. & Kaufman, F.R. (1994) Androgen and the development of human sex-typical behavior: rough-and-tumble play and sex of preferred playmates in children with congenital adrenal hyperplasia (CAH). *Child Dev.*, **65**, 1042–1053.

Honda, S., Harada, N., Ito, S., Takagi, Y. & Maeda, S. (1998) Disruption of sexual behavior in male aromatase-deficient mice lacking exons 1 and 2 of the cyp19 gene. *Biochem. Biophys. Res. Commun.*, **252**, 445–449.

Houtsmuller, E.J., Brand, T., de Jonge, F.H., Joosten, R.N., van de Poll, N.E. & Slob, A.K. (1994) SDN-POA volume, sexual behavior, and partner preference of male rats affected by perinatal treatment with ATD. *Physiol. Behav.*, **56**, 535–541.

Hu, S., Pattatucci, A.M., Patterson, C., Li, L., Fulker, D.W., Cherny, S.S., Kruglyak, L. & Hamer, D.H. (1995) Linkage between sexual orientation and chromosome Xq28 in males but not in females. *Nat. Genet.*, **11**, 248–256.

Hyde, J.S., Lindberg, S.M., Linn, M.C., Ellis, A.B. & Williams, C.C. (2008) Diversity. Gender similarities characterize math performance. *Science*, **321**, 494–495.

Iijima, M., Arisaka, O., Minamoto, F. & Arai, Y. (2001) Sex differences in children's free drawings: a study on girls with congenital adrenal hyperplasia. *Horm. Behav.*, **40**, 99–104.

Imperato-McGinley, J. (1994) 5 alpha-reductase deficiency: human and animal models. *Eur. Eurol.*, **25** Suppl 1, 20–23.

Imperato-McGinley, J., Miller, M., Wilson, J.D., Peterson, R.E., Shackleton, C. & Gajdusek, D.C. (1991) A cluster of male pseudohermaphrodites with 5 alpha-reductase deficiency in Papua New Guinea. *Clin. Endocrinol. (Oxf)*, **34**, 293–298.

Imperato-McGinley, J. & Zhu, Y.S. (2002) Androgens and male physiology the syndrome of 5alpha-reductase-2 deficiency. *Mol. Cell. Endocrinol.*, **198**, 51–59.

Imwalle, D.B., Bateman, H.L., Wills, A., Honda, S., Harada, N. & Rissman, E.F. (2006) Impairment of spatial learning by estradiol treatment in female mice is attenuated by estradiol exposure during development. *Horm. Behav.*, **50**, 693–698.

Jacobson, C.D., Csernus, V.J., Shryne, J.E. & Gorski, R.A. (1981) The influence of gonadectomy, androgen exposure, or a gonadal graft in the neonatal rat on the volume of the sexually dimorphic nucleus of the preoptic area. *J. Neurosci.*, **1**, 1142–1147.

Jacobson, C.D., Shryne, J.E., Shapiro, F. & Gorski, R.A. (1980) Ontogeny of the sexually dimorphic nucleus of the preoptic area. *J. Comp Neurol.*, **193**, 541–548.

Jimbo, M., Okubo, K., Toma, Y., Shimizu, Y., Saito, H. & Yanaihara, T. (1998) Inhibitory effects of catecholamines and maternal stress on aromatase activity in the fetal rat brain. *J. Obstet. Gynaecol. Res.*, **24**, 291–297.

Katz, J.N. (1976) *Gay American History: Lesbians and Gay Men in the U.S.A.* T.Y. Crowell, New York.

Kelley, D.B. & Pfaff, D.W. (1978) Generalizations from comparative studies on neuroanatomical and endocrine mechanisms of sexual behaviour. In Hutchison, J.B. (ed) *Biological determinants of sexual behaviour.* John Wiley & Sons, Chichester, pp. 225–254.

Kerchner, M. & Ward, I.L. (1992) SDN-MPOA volume in male rats is decreased by prenatal stress, but is not related to ejaculatory behavior. *Brain Res.*, **581**, 244–251.

Kessler, S.J. & McKenna, W. (1978) *Gender: an ethno-methodological approach.* Wiley, New York.

Keverne, E.B. (1999) The vomeronasal organ. *Science*, **286**, 716–720.

Kinsey, A.C., Pomeroy, W.R. & Martin, C.E. (1948) *Sexual behavior in the human male.* W.B. Saunders Company, Philadelphia.

Kinsey, A.C., Pomeroy, W.R., Martin, C.E. & Gebhard, P.H. (1953) *Sexual behavior in the human female.* Saunders, Philadelphia.

Kiumura, D. (1999) *Sex and cognition.* MIT Press, Cambridge.

Kourany, R.F. (1987) Suicide among homosexual adolescents. *J. Homosex.*, **13**, 111–117.

Kraemer, B., Noll, T., Delsignore, A., Milos, G., Schnyder, U. & Hepp, U. (2006) Finger length ratio (2D:4D) and dimensions of sexual orientation. *Neuropsychobiology*, **53**, 210–214.

Kruijver, F.P.M., Balesar, R., Espila, A.M., Unmehopa, U.A. & Swaab, D.F. (2002) Estrogen receptor-alpha distribution in the human hypothalamus in relation to sex and endocrine status. *J. Comp. Neurol.*, **454**, 115–139.

Kruijver, F.P.M., Balesar, R., Espila, A.M., Unmehopa, U.A. & Swaab, D.F. (2003) Estrogen-receptor-beta distribution in the human hypothalamus: Similarities and differences with ERalpha distribution. *J. Comp. Neurol.*, **466**, 251–277.

Kruijver, F.P.M., de Jonge, F.H., van den Broek, W.T., van der Woude, T., Endert, E. & Swaab, D.F. (1993) Lesions of the suprachiasmatic nucleus do not disturb sexual orientation of the adult male rat. *Brain Res.*, **624**, 342–346.

Kruijver, F.P.M., Fernández-Guasti, A., Fodor, M., Kraan, E.M. & Swaab, D.F. (2001) Sex differences in androgen receptors of the human mamillary bodies are related to endocrine status rather than to sexual orientation or transsexuality. *J. Clin. Endocrinol. Metab.*, **86**, 818–827.

Lalumiere, M.L., Blanchard, R. & Zucker, K.J. (2000) Sexual orientation and handedness in men and women: a meta-analysis. *Psychol. Bull*, **126**, 575–592.

Lebson, M. (2002) Suicide among homosexual youth. *J. Homosex.*, **42**, 107–117.

Legros, J.J., Van Cauwenberge, H., Lambotte, R., Bauduin, A., Franchimont, P. & Legros, J. (1974) Problèmes psycho-endocriniens posés par un cas d'hyperplasie surrénalienne congénitale reconnu tardivement. *Revue Médicale de Liège*, **29**, 73–80.

LeVay, S. (1991) A difference in hypothalamic structure between heterosexual and homosexual men. *Science*, **253**, 1034–1037.

LeVay, S. (1993) *The sexual brain.* MIT Press, Cambridge, MA.

LeVay, S. (1996) *Queer science.* MIT Press, Cambridge, MA.

LeVay, S. (2010) *Gay, straight, and the reason why. The science of sexual orientation.* Oxford University Press, New York.

LeVay, S. & Hamer, D.H. (1994) Evidence for a biological influence in male homosexuality. *Sci. Am.*, **270**, 44–49.

LeVay, S. & Valente, S.M. (2006) *Human Sexuallity.* Sinauer Associates Inc, Sunderland, MA.

Lippa, R.A. (2003a) Are 2D:4D finger-length ratios related to sexual orientation? Yes for men, no for women. *J. Pers. Soc. Psychol.*, **85**, 179–188.

Lippa, R.A. (2003b) Handedness, sexual orientation, and gender-related personality traits in men and women. *Arch. Sex. Behav.*, **32**, 103–114.

Lorenz, K. (1937) Uber die Bildung des Instinktbergiffes (The establishment of the instinct concept). *Die Naturwissenschaften*, **25**, 280–300, 307–318, 325–331.

Lorenz, K. (1950) The comparative method in studying innate behavior patterns. *Symp. Soc. Exp. Biol.*, **4**, 221–268.

Lutchmaya, S., Baron-Cohen, S. & Raggatt, P. (2002) Foetal testosterone and eye contact in 12-month-old human infants. *Infant Behav. Develop*, **25**, 327–335.

Lutchmaya, S., Baron-Cohen, S., Raggatt, P., Knickmeyer, R. & Manning, J.T. (2004) 2nd to 4th digit ratios, fetal testosterone and estradiol. *Early Hum. Dev.*, **77**, 23–28.

MacLaughlin, D.T. & Donahoe, P.K. (2004) Sex determination and differentiation. *N. Engl. J. Med.*, **350**, 367–378.

Manning, J.T., Fink, B., Neave, N. & Szwed, A. (2006) The second to fourth digit ratio and asymmetry. *Ann. Hum. Biol.*, **33**, 480–492.

Mansukhani, V., Adkins-Regan, E. & Yang, S. (1996) Sexual partner preference in female zebra finches: The role of early hormones and social environment. *Horm. Behav.*, **30**, 506–513.

Marler, P. & Hamilton, W.J.I. (1966) *Mechanisms of animal behavior.* Wiley and Sons, New York.

Martin, J.T. & Nguyen, D.H. (2004) Anthropometric analysis of homosexuals and heterosexuals: implications for early hormone exposure. *Horm. Behav.*, **45**, 31–39.

McCormick, C.M. & Witelson, S.F. (1991) A cognitive profile of homosexual men compared to heterosexual men and women. *Psychoneuroendocrinology*, **16**, 459–73.

McEwen, B.S. & Alves, S.E. (1999) Estrogen actions in the central nervous system. *Endocr. Rev.*, **20**, 279–307.

McFadden, D. (2002) Masculinization effects in the auditory system. *Arch. Sex. Behav.*, **31**, 99–111.

McFadden, D. (2008) What do sex, twins, spotted hyenas, ADHD, and sexual orientation have in common? *Perspectives Psychol. Sci*, **3**, 309–323.

McFadden, D. (2011) Sexual orientation and the auditory system. *Front. Neuroendocrinol.*, **32**, 201–213.

McFadden, D. & Champlin, C.A. (2000) Comparison of auditory evoked potentials in heterosexual, homosexual, and bisexual males and females. *J. Assoc. Res. Otolaryngol.*, **1**, 89–99.

McFadden, D. & Pasanen, E.G. (1998) Comparison of the auditory systems of heterosexuals and homosexuals: click-evoked otoacoustic emissions. *Proc. Natl. Acad. Sci. U S A*, **95**, 2709–2713.

McFadden, D. & Pasanen, E.G. (1999) Spontaneous otoacoustic emissions in hetero-sexuals, homosexuals, and bisexuals. *J. Acoust. Soc. Am.*, **105**, 2403–2413.

McFadden, D., Pasanen, E.G., Valero, M.D., Roberts, E.K. & Lee, T.M. (2009) Effect of prenatal androgens on click-evoked otoacoustic emissions in male and female sheep (Ovis aries). *Horm. Behav.*, **55**, 98–105.

McFadden, D. & Shubel, E. (2002) Relative lengths of fingers and toes in human males and females. *Horm. Behav.,* **42**, 492–500.

Meredith, M. (2001) Human vomeronasal organ function: a critical review of best and worst cases. *Chem. Senses*, **26**, 433–445.

Meyer-Bahlburg, H.F. (1984) Psychoendocrine research on sexual orientation. Current status and future options. *Prog. Brain Res.,* **61**, 375–398.

Meyer-Bahlburg, H.F. (2005) Gender identity outcome in female-raised 46, XY persons with penile agenesis, cloacal exstrophy of the bladder, or penile ablation. *Arch. Sex. Behav.*, **34**, 423–438.

Meyer-Bahlburg, H.F. (2009) Male Gender Identity in an XX Individual with Congenital Adrenal Hyperplasia. *J. Sex. Med.* 5, 298–299.

Meyer-Bahlburg, H.F., Dolezal, C., Baker, S.W. & New, M.I. (2008) Sexual orientation in women with classical or non-classical congenital adrenal hyperplasia as a function of degree of prenatal androgen excess. *Arch. Sex. Behav.,* **37**, 85–99.

Meyer-Bahlburg, H.F., Ehrhardt, A.A. & Rosen, L.R. (1995) Prenatal estrogens and the development of homosexual orientation. *Dev. Psychol.*, **s31**, 12–21.

Micevych, P. & Dominguez, R. (2009) Membrane estradiol signaling in the brain. *Front. Neuroendocrinol.*, **30**, 315–327.

Miller, G. (2008) Neuroimaging. Growing pains for fMRI. *Science*, **320**, 1412–1414.

Miller, G., Tybur, J. & Jordan, B.D. (2007) Ovulatory cycle effects on tip earnings by lap dancers: economic evidence for human estrus? *Evolution and Human Behavior*, **28**, 375–381.

Money, J. & Ehrhardt, A.A. (1972) *Man & Woman, Boy & Girl.* Johns Hopkins University Press, Baltimore.

Money, J., Schwartz, M. & Lewis, V.G. (1984) Adult erotosexual status and fetal hor-monal masculinization and demasculinization: 46, XX congenital virilizing adrenal hyperplasia and 46, XY androgen-insensitivity syndrome compared. *Psychoneuroen-docrinology*, **9**, 405–414.

Morrell, J.I. & Pfaff, D.W. (1978) A neuroendocrine approach to brain function: localization of sex steroid concentrating cells in vertebrate brains. *Amer. Zool.*, **18**, 447–460.

Mosher, W.D., Chandra, A. & Jones, J. (2005) Sexual behavior and selected health mea-sures: men and women 15–44 years of age, United States 2002. http://www.cdc/gov/nchs/data/ad/ad362.pdf.

Mustanski, B.S., Dupree, M.G., Nievergelt, C.M., Bocklandt, S., Schork, N.J. & Hamer, D.H. (2005) A genomewide scan of male sexual orientation. *Hum. Genet.*, **116**, 272–278.

Nardi, P. (1992) *Men's friendships.* Sage Publications, Newbury Park, CA.

Neave, N., Menaged, M. & Weightman, D.R. (1999) Sex differences in cognition: the role of testosterone and sexual orientation. *Brain Cogn.*, **41**, 245–262.

Nelson, R.J. (2005) *An introduction to behavioral endocrinology.* Sinauer Associates, Inc., Sunderland, Massachussets.

Ngun, T.C., Ghahramani, N., Sanchez, F.J., Bocklandt, S. & Vilain, E. (2011) The genetics of sex differences in brain and behavior. *Front. Neuroendocrinol.*, **32**, 227–246.

Nordenstrom, A., Servin, A., Bohlin, G., Larsson, A. & Wedell, A. (2002) Sex-typed toy play behavior correlates with the degree of prenatal androgen exposure assessed by CYP21 genotype in girls with congenital adrenal hyperplasia. *J. Clin. Endocrinol. Metab.*, **87**, 5119–5124.

Nottebohm, F. & Arnold, A.P. (1976) Sexual dimorphism in vocal control areas of the songbird brain. *Science*, **194**, 211–213.

Onfray, M. (2010) *Le crépuscule d'une idole. L'affabulation freudienne.* Bernard Grasset, Paris.

Op de Beeck, H.P., Haushofer, J. & Kanwisher, N.G. (2008) Interpreting fMRI data: maps, modules and dimensions. *Nat. Rev. Neurosci.*, **9**, 123–135.

Ozdemir, S.T., Ercan, I., Sevinc, O., Guney, I., Ocakoglu, G., Aslan, E. & Barut, C. (2007) Statistical shape analysis of differences in the shape of the corpus callosum between genders. *Anat. Rec. (Hoboken)*, **290**, 825–830.

Paredes, R.G. & Baum, M.J. (1995) Altered sexual partner preference in male ferrets given excitotoxic lesions of the preoptic area anterior hypothalamus. *J. Neurosci.*, **15**, 6619–6630.

Paredes, R.G., Tzschentke, T. & Nakach, N. (1998) Lesions of the medial preoptic area anterior hypothalamus (MPOA/AH) modify partner preference in male rats. *Brain Res.*, **813**, 1–8.

Pelletier, G. (2000) Localization of androgen and estrogen receptors in rat and primate tissues. *Histol. Histopathol.*, **15**, 1261–1270.

Perkins, A. & Fitzgerald, J.A. (1992) Luteinizing hormone, testosterone, and behavioral response of male-oriented rams to estrous ewes and rams. *J. Anim. Sci.*, **70**, 1787–1794.

Perkins, A., Fitzgerald, J.A. & Price, E.O. (1992) Luteinizing hormone and testosterone response of sexually active and inactive rams. *J. Anim. Sci.*, **70**, 2086–2093.

Perkins, A. & Roselli, C.E. (2007) The ram as a model for behavioral neuroendocrinology. *Horm. Behav.*, **52**, 70–77.

Pinckard, K.L., Stellflug, J., Resko, J.A., Roselli, C.E. & Stormshak, F. (2000) Review: brain aromatization and other factors affecting male reproductive behavior with emphasis on the sexual orientation of rams. *Domes. Anim. Endocrinol.*, **18**, 83–96.

Poianni, A. (2010) *Animal homosexuality. A biological perspective.* Cambridge University Press, Cambridge UK.

Rahman, Q., Abrahams, S. & Wilson, G.D. (2003a) Sexual-orientation-related differences in verbal fluency. *Neuropsychology*, **17**, 240–246.

Rahman, Q., Kumari, V. & Wilson, G.D. (2003b) Sexual orientation-related differences in prepulse inhibition of the human startle response. *Behav. Neurosci.*, **117**, 1096–1102.

Rahman, Q. & Wilson, G.D. (2003a) Born gay? The psychobiology of human sexual orientation. *Personality and Individual Differences*, **34**, 1337–1382.

Rahman, Q. & Wilson, G.D. (2003b) Large sexual-orientation-related differences in performance on mental rotation and judgment of line orientation tasks. *Neuropsychology*, **17**, 25–31.

Rahman, Q. & Wilson, G.D. (2003c) Sexual orientation and the 2nd to 4th finger length ratio: evidence for organising effects of sex hormones or developmental instability? *Psychoneuroendocrinology*, **28**, 288–303.

Raisman, G. & Field, P.M. (1971) Sexual dimorphism in the preoptic area of the rat. *Science*, **173**, 731–733.

Reiner, W.G. & Gearhart, J.P. (2004) Discordant sexual identity in some genetic males with cloacal exstrophy assigned to female sex at birth. *N. Engl. J. Med.*, **350**, 333–341.

Resko, J.A., Perkins, A., Roselli, C.E., Fitzgerald, J.A., Choate, J.V. & Stormshak, F. (1996) Endocrine correlates of partner preference behavior in rams. *Biol. Reprod.*, **55**, 120–126.

Rhees, R.W., Shryne, J.E. & Gorski, R.A. (1990) Termination of the hormone-sensitive period for differentiation of the sexually dimorphic nucleus of the preoptic area in male and female rats. *Dev. Brain Res.*, **52**, 17–23.

Rice, G., Anderson, C., Risch, N. & Ebers, G. (1999) Male homosexuality: absence of linkage to microsatellite markers at Xq28. *Science*, **284**, 665–667.

Richelle, M. (1966) *Le conditionnement operant.* Delachaux et Niestlé, Neuchatel, Suisse.

Rieger, G., Chivers, M.L. & Bailey, J.M. (2005) Sexual arousal patterns of bisexual men. *Psychol. Sci*, **16**, 579–584.

Robarts, D.W & Baum, M.J. (2007) Ventromedial hypothalamic nucleus lesions disrupt olfactory mate recognition and receptivity in female ferrets. *Horm. Behav.*, **51**, 104–113.

Romano, M., Rubolini, D., Martinelli, R., Bonisoli Alquati, A. & Saino, N. (2005) Experimental manipulation of yolk testosterone affects digit length ratios in the ring-necked pheasant (Phasianus colchicus). *Horm. Behav.*, **48**, 342–346.

Roselli, C.E., Larkin, K., Resko, J.A., Stellflug, J.N. & Stormshak, F. (2004a) The volume of a sexually dimorphic nucleus in the ovine medial preoptic area/anterior hypothalamus varies with sexual partner preference. *Endocrinology*, **145**, 478–483.

Roselli, C.E., Larkin, K., Schrunk, J.M. & Stormshak, F. (2004b) Sexual partner preference, hypothalamic morphology and aromatase in rams. *Physiol. Behav.*, **83**, 233–245.

Roselli, C.E., Reddy, R. & Kaufman, K. (2011) The development of male-oriented behavior in rams. *Front. Neuroendocrinol.* 32, 164–169

Roselli, C.E., Stadelman, H., Reeve, R., Bishop, C.V. & Stormshak, F. (2007) The ovine sexually dimorphic nucleus of the medial preoptic area is organized prenatally by testosterone. *Endocrinology*, **148**, 4450–4457.

Rosenzweig, M.R., Breedlove, S.M. & Watson, N.V. (2004) *Biological psychology: An introduction to behavioral and cognitive neuroscience.* Sinauer Associates, Sunderland MA.

Rosler, A. & Witztum, E. (1998) Treatment of men with paraphilia with a long-acting analogue of gonadotropin-releasing hormone. *N. Engl. J. Med.*, **338**, 416–422.

Rubin, R.T., Reinisch, J.M. & Haskett, R.F. (1981) Postnatal gonadal steroid effects on human behavior. *Science*, **211**, 1318–1324.

Sanders, A.R. & Dawood, K. (2003) *Nature encyclopedia of life sciences.* Nature Publishing Group, London.

Savic, I., Berglund, H., Gulyas, B. & Roland, P. (2001) Smelling of odorous sex hormone-like compounds causes sex-differentiated hypothalamic activations in humans. *Neuron*, **31**, 661–668.

Savic, I., Berglund, H. & Lindstrom, P. (2005) Brain response to putative pheromones in homosexual men. *Proc. Natl. Acad. Sci. U S A*, **102**, 7356–7361.

Schmidt, G. & Clement, U. (1990) Does peace prevent homosexuality? *Arch. Sex. Behav.*, **19**, 183–187.

Schober, J.M., Carmichael, P.A., Hines, M. & Ransley, P.G. (2002) The ultimate challenge of cloacal exstrophy. *J. Urol.*, **167**, 300–304.

Sherwin, B.B. & Gelfand, M.M. (1987) The role of androgen in the maintenance of sexual functioning in oophorectomized women. *Psychosom. Med.*, **49**, 397–409.

Sinclair, A.H., Berta, P., Palmer, M.S., Hawkins, J.R., Griffiths, B.L., Smith, M.J., Foster, J.W., Frischauf, A.M., Lovell-Badge, R. & Goodfellow, P.N. (1990) A gene from the human sex-determining region encodes a protein with homology to a conserved DNA-binding motif. *Nature*, **346**, 240–244.

Sisk, C.L. & Zehr, J.L. (2005) Pubertal hormones organize the adolescent brain and behavior. *Front. Neuroendocrinol.*, **26**, 163–174.

Skinner, B.F. (1965) *L'analyse expérimentale du comportement*. Pierre Mardaga, Wavre.

Skinner, B.F. (1971) *L'analyse expérimentale du comportement (Traduit de l'Amércain par A.M et M. Richelle)*. Charles Dessart, Bruxelles.

Snyder, P.J., Peachey, H., Berlin, J.A., Hannoush, P., Haddad, G., Dlewati, A., Santanna, J., Loh, L., Lenrow, D.A., Holmes, J.H., Kapoor, S.C., Atkinson, L.E. & Strom, B.L. (2000) Effects of testosterone replacement in hypogonadal men. *J. Clin. Endocrinol. Metab.*, **85**, 2670–2677.

Sommer, V. & Vasey, P.L. (2006) *Homosexual behaviour in animals. An evolutionary perspective*. Cambridge University Press, Cambridge.

Stacey, J. & Biblarz, T.J. (2001) (How) does the sexual orientation of parents matter? *American Sociological Review*, **66**, 159–183.

Strong, B. & DeVault, C. (1997) *Human sexuality*. Mayfield Publishing Co, Mountain View, CA.

Swaab, D.F. (2007) Sexual differentiation of the brain and behavior. *Best Pract. Res. Clin. Endocrinol. Metab.*, **21**, 431–444.

Swaab, D.F. & Fliers, E. (1985) A sexually dimorphic nucleus in the human brain. *Science*, **228**, 1112–1115.

Swaab, D.F. & Hofman, M.A. (1988) Sexual differentiation of the human hypothalamus: Ontogeny of the sexually dimorphic nucleus of the preoptic area. *Dev. Brain Res.*, **44**, 314–318.

Swaab, D.F. & Hofman, M.A. (1990) An enlarged suprachiasmatic nucleus in homosexual men. *Brain Res.*, **537**, 141–148.

Taziaux, M., Keller, M., Bakker, J. & Balthazart, J. (2007) Sexual behavior activity tracks rapid changes in brain estrogen concentrations. *J. Neurosci.*, **27**, 6563–6572.

Titus-Ernstoff, L., Perez, K., Hatch, E.E., Troisi, R., Palmer, J.R., Hartge, P., Hyer, M., Kaufman, R., Adam, E., Strohsnitter, W., Noller, K., Pickett, K.E. & Hoover, R. (2003) Psychosexual characteristics of men and women exposed prenatally to diethylstilbestrol. *Epidemiology*, **14**, 155–160.

Tuncer, M.C., Hatipoglu, E.S. & Ozates, M. (2005) Sexual dimorphism and handedness in the human corpus callosum based on magnetic resonance imaging. *Surg. Radiol. Anat.*, **27**, 254–259.

Tutle, G.E. & Pillard, R.C. (1991) Sexual orientation and cognitive abilities. *Arch. Sex. Behav.*, **20**, 307–318.

Udry, J.R., Billy, J.O., Morris, N.M., Groff, T.R. & Raj, M.H. (1985) Serum androgenic hormones motivate sexual behavior in adolescent boys. *Fertil. Steril.*, **43**, 90–94.

Van Rillaer, J. (1980) *Les illusions de la psychanalyse*. Pierre Mardaga, Sprimont (Belgique).

Vasudevan, N. & Pfaff, D.W. (2008) Non-genomic actions of estrogens and their inter-action with genomic actions in the brain. *Front. Neuroendocrinol.*, **29**, 238–257.

Vermeulen, A., Rubens, R. & Verdonck, L. (1972) Testosterone secretion and metabolism in male senescence. *J. Clin. Endocrinol. Metab.*, **34**, 730–735.

Vidal, C. (ed) (2000) *Féminin Masculin Mythes et idéologie*. Belin, Paris.

Vidal, C. (2007) *Hommes, femmes avons-nous le même cerveau?* Le Pommier, Paris.

Wallen, K. (2009) Does finger fat produce sex differences in second to fourth digit ratios? *Endocrinology*, **150**, 4819–4822.

Wang, C., Swerdloff, R.S., Iranmanesh, A., Dobs, A., Snyder, P.J., Cunningham, G., Matsumoto, A.M., Weber, T., Berman, N. & Grp, T.G.S. (2000) Transdermal testosterone gel improves sexual function, mood, muscle strength, and body composition parameters in hypogonadal men. *J. Clin. Endocrinol. Metab.*, **85**, 2839–2853.

Ward, I.L. (1972) Prenatal stress feminizes and demasculinizes the behavior of males. *Science*, **175**, 82–84.

Ward, I.L. (1984) The prenatal stress syndrome: current status. *Psychoneuroendocrinology*, **9**, 3–11.

Ward, I.L. & Ward, O.B. (1985) Sexual behavior differentiation: effects of prenatal manipulations in rats *Handbook of Behavioral Neurobiology, Reproduction.* 7, 77–98.

Weisz, J. (1983) Influence of maternal stress on the developmental pattern of the steroidogenic function in Leydig cells and steroid aromatase activity in the brain of rat fetuses. *Monogr. Neural. Sci.*, **9**, 184–193.

Wellings, K., Field, J., Johnson, A.M. & Wadsworth, J. (1994) *Sexual behavior in Britain: The National Survey of Sexual Attitudes and Lifestyles*. Penguin Books, London.

Williams, C.L. & Pleil, K.E. (2008) Toy story: why do monkey and human males prefer trucks? Comment on "Sex differences in rhesus monkey toy preferences parallel those of children" by Hassett, Siebert and Wallen. *Horm. Behav.*, **54**, 355–358.

Wisniewski, A.B., Migeon, C.J., Meyer-Bahlburg, H.F., Gearhart, J.P., Berkovitz, G.D., Brown, T.R. & Money, J. (2000) Complete androgen insensitivity syndrome: long-term medical, surgical, and psychosexual outcome. *J. Clin. Endocrinol. Metab.*, **85**, 2664–2669.

Witelson, S.F., Kigar, D.L., Scamvougeras, A., Kideckel, D.M., Buck, B., Stanchev, P.L., Bronskill, M. & Black, S. (2008) Corpus Callosum Anatomy in Right-Handed Homosexual and Heterosexual Men. *Arch. Sex. Behav.* 37, 857–863

Wysocki, C.J. & Preti, G. (2004) Facts, fallacies, fears, and frustrations with human pheromones. *Anat. Rec. A Discov. Mol. Cell. Evol. Biol.*, **281**, 1201–1211.

Yang, X., Schadt, E.E., Wang, S., Wang, H., Arnold, A.P., Ingram-Drake, L., Drake, T.A. & Lusis, A.J. (2006) Tissue-specific expression and regulation of sexually dimorphic genes in mice. *Genome Res.*, **16**, 995–1004.

Zhou, J.N., Hofman, M.A., Gooren, L.J.G. & Swaab, D.F. (1995) A sex difference in the human brain and its relation to transsexuality. *Nature*, **378**, 68–70.

Zucker, K.J., Bradley, S.J., Oliver, G., Blake, J., Fleming, S. & Hood, J. (1996) Psycho-sexual development of women with congenital adrenal hyperplasia. *Horm. Behav.*, **30**, 300–318.

Index